Get Your Health Back with Alternative Medicines

Major Fred Martin

Get Your Health Back with Alternative Medicines
Copyright © 2023 by Major Fred Martin

All rights reserved. No part of this publication may be reproduced, distributed, or transmitted in any form or by any means, including photocopying, recording, or other electronic or mechanical methods, without the prior written permission of the author, except in the case of brief quotations embodied in critical reviews and certain other non-commercial uses permitted by copyright law.

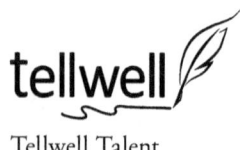

Tellwell Talent
www.tellwell.ca

ISBN
978-0-2288-8640-2 (Hardcover)
978-0-2288-8639-6 (Paperback)
978-0-2288-8641-9 (eBook)

INTEGUMENTARY SYSTEM:

An aggregation of tissue that performs a specific function is an organ - next highest level of organisation is a system. A group of organs performing together to perform specific functions - the skin - hair - nails - glands - also several specialised receptors make up the **integumentary system.** The skin is quite complex in structure - performing several functions essential for survival. The skin of an average human adult, covers $2m^2$, the largest organ in terms of surface area of the human body.

physiology:

there are numerous functions of the skin.

[1] regulates the body temperature:

in response to high environmental temperatures, or strenuous exercise - the production of perspiration by sudoriferous glands helps in normalising body temperature – changes to the skins blood flow - also alters its insulating properties - helping to adjust body temperature.

[2] protection:

the skin covering provides a physical barrier protecting the underlying tissues from physical damage - bacterial invasion - dehydration - and ultraviolet radiation - UV.

[3] reception of stimuli:

the skin contains numerous nerve endings and receptors which detect stimuli - relating to touch - temperature - pain and pressure.

[4] excretion:

perspiration not only helps in regulating normal body temperature - it assists in excretion of tiny amounts of water - salts - several organic compounds - and toxic waste.

[5] **synthesis of vitamin** D:

The terminology, **vitamin** D, refers to a group of closely related compounds which are synthesised naturally from a precursor molecule present in the skin when exposed to ultraviolet radiation [UV].

<u>In the skin;</u>
precursor substance, 7-dehydrocholesterol, converted to cholecalciferol **vitamin** D_3 in the presence of UV.

<u>In the liver;</u>
cholecalciferol is converted to **25**-hydroxycholecalciferol.

<u>In the kidneys;</u>
this substance is changed into **1,25**-dihydroxycalciferol (**calcitriol**), most active form of vitamin D which stimulates the absorption of **calcium** and **phosphorus** from dietary foods - **vitamin** D is actually a **hormone,** produced in one area of the body (the abdomen) - transported by the blood - then it exerts its effect to another location.

HOMEOSTATIC IMBALANCES of the INTEGUMENTARY SYSTEM: (part one) 58

abrasions	abscess	acne	actinic keratosis	ageing skin
athletes foot	baldness	bites	blepharitis	blisters
boils - carbuncles	bruising	burns	callous	chicken pox
cellular tissue damage	chilblains	cold sores	comedo	conjunctivitis
corns	dandruff	decubitus ulcers	eczema	elasticity-skin
elephantiasis	erythema	german measles	herpes	hives
hydration-skin	impetigo	insect-bites	odour	papule
pediculosis	perspiration	phlebitis	pruritis	psoriasis
scabies	scarring	scleroderma	seborrhoea	sebum
shingles	snake-bites	stretchmarks	sunburn	sun-tanning
surface-veins	s-l-erythematosus	tinea	urticaria	warts
windburn	wounds	x-rays.		

THERAPEUTIC ACTIONS for the INTEGUMENTARY IMBALANCES: (part two) 56

antiageing	antiallergenics	antibiotics	antifungal	anti-inflammatant
antipruritic	antisclerotics	antiscorbutic	antiseptic	antisudorific
antivenomous	antiviral	arterial vaso-dilator	astringents	bactericidal

bacteriostatic	cicatrisant	cobalt therapy	collagen treatment	cytophylactic
deodourant	disinfectant	emollient	eye-muscle-strengthener escharotics	
facial-capillary-treat	haemostatic	hair-growth-stimulant	hair tonic	hydrating-essence
hypersensitivity	insecticide	insect repellents	parasiticide	penetrating-oil
photo-toxic	preservative	prophylactic	radiation-antidote	rejuvenator-skin
rehydration	resolvent	rubefacient	skin cleanser	skin-glands
skin-photo-sensitisation	skin-tone	skin-types	styptic	sudorific
tissue stimulant	vasoconstrictor	vasodilator	venous-tonic	vulnerary
weight loss.				

THERAPEUTIC ESSENCES for the INTEGUMENTARY IMBALANCES: (part three) 79

[s] amyris	[**st**] angelica root	[**st**] aniseed	[**st**] swt basil	[**st**] bay laurel
[s] benzoin	[s] bergamot	[**st**] birch bud	[**st**] black pepper	[s] brahmi
[**st**] cajeputi	[**st**] caraway seed	[**st**] carrot seed	[s] cedarwood atlas	[s] celery seed
[s] chamomiles	[**st**] cinnamon leaf	[s] clary sage	[**st**] clove bud	[**st**] coriander
[s] cypress	[**st**] elemi	[**st**] eucalyptus radiata	[**st**] swt fennel seed	[s] fir needle

[s] frankencense	[**st**] galbanum	[**st**] garlic	[**n**] geranium	[**st**] ginger
[**st**] grapefruit	[s] guaiacwood	[s] helichrysum	[s] hypericum	[**st**] hyssop
[s] immortelle	[**st**] inula	[s] jasmine	[**st**] juniper berry	[**st**] lavandin
[s] lavender	[**st**] spike lavender	[**n**] lemon	[**st**] lemongrass	[**n**] lime
[s] linden blossom	[s] mandarin	[s] swt marjoram	[**st**] may chang	[s] melissa
[**st**] myrrh	[**n**] myrtle	[s] neroli	[**st**] niaouli	[s] swt orange
[**st**] origanum	[**st**] palmarosa	[**st**] parsley herb	[s] patchouli	[**st**] peppermint
[s] pettitgrain	[**st**] pimento leaf	[**st**] pine needles.	[**st**] rose geranium	[s] rose
[**st**] rosemary	[**st**] rosewood	[s] sandalwood	[**st**] spearmint	[s] spikenard
[s] tagetes	[s] tangerine	[**st**] tea tree	[**st**] swt thyme	[s] verbena
[s] vetivert	[s] violet leaf	[**st**] yarrow	[s] ylang-ylang.	

HOMEOSTATIC IMBALANCES for the INTEGUMENTARY SYSTEM: (part one) 60

abrasions	abscess	acne	actinic keratosis	ageing skin
athletes foot	baldness	bites	blepharitis	blisters
boils - carbuncles	bruising	burns	callous	chicken pox
cellular tissue damage	chilblains	cold sores	comedo	conjunctivitis

corns	dandruff	decubitus ulcers	eczema	elasticity-skin
elephantiasis	erythema	german measles	herpes	hives
hydration-skin	impetigo	insect-bites	odour	papule
pediculosis	perspiration	phlebitis	pruritis	psoriasis
scabies	scarring	scleroderma	seborrhoea	sebum
shingles	snake-bites	stretchmarks	sunburn	sun-tanning
surface-veins	s-l-erythematosus	tinea	urticaria	warts
windburn	wounds	x-rays.		

---

abrasions:
A portion of skin which has been removed by injuries etc, ie; scraping.
All pure essential plant essences inhibit the **growth** of **organisms, bacteria** and **germs**.

antiseptic-essences:
helps in the **prevention** of **tissue degeneration** - also in the controlling of infections.

[s] amyris	[**st**] bay laurel	[s] benzoin	[s]***bergamot**
[**n**] birch bud	[**st**] black pepper	[**st**] cajeputi	[**st**] caraway seed
[s] cedarwood atlas	[s] german chamomile	[s] roman chamomile	[**st**] cinnamon leaf
[s] clary sage	[**st**] clove bud	[**st**] cumin	[s] cypress
[**st**]***eucalyptus radiata**	[**st**] swt fennel seed	[s] fir needle	[s]***frankincense**
[**n**] geranium	[**st**] ginger	[**st**] grapefruit	[s]***helichrysum**
[**b**] hyssop	[s] jasmine	[**st**]***juniper berry**	[**st**] lavandin
[s]***lavender**	[**st**] spike lavender	[**n**] lemon	[s] lemongrass

[n] lime	[s] swt marjoram	[st] may chang	[st] myrrh (thyroid)
[n] myrtle	[st] niaouli	[st] nutmeg	[s] swt orange
[st] origanum	[st] palmarosa	[s] parsley herb	[s] patchouli
[st]*peppermint	[st] pine needles	[s] rose	[st] rose geranium
[st]*rosemary	[s] rosewood	[s]*sandalwood	[st] spikenard
[s] tagetes	[s] tangerine	[st]*tea tree	[st] swt thyme
[s] verbena, lemon	[s] vetivert	[s] violet leaf	[st] yarrow
[s] ylang-ylang…			

<u>excretory-antiseptic</u>: [st]***juniper berry**.

---

abscess:
a localised collection of pus and liquefied tissue in a cavity - an abcess in usually treated in Aromatherapy by means of hot compresses placed over the swelling to reduce pain and inflammation; to **draw out** toxic matter - by using **anti-inflammatant-agents**.

<u>anti-inflammatant-essences</u>:
reduce the pain and swelling of inflammation.

[s]***ammi visnaga**	[s]***amyris**	[st]***angelica root**	[st]***artemesia** arborescens
[s]***bergamot**	[n]***calendula**	[st]***cedarwood atlas**	[s] celery seed
[s]***chamomiles**	[s] clary sage	[st]***eucalyptus rad**	[st]***swt fennel seed**
[s] guaiacwood	[s] helichrysum	[s] immortelle	[s] inula
[s]***lavender**	[st]***myrrh**	[s] patchouli	[st]***peppermint**
[st] pine needles	[s] rose	[s] sandalwood	[st] santolina
[s] tagetes	[st] turmeric	[st] yarrow.	
[st]***swt fennel seed**;	(prevents **toxic waste build-up** in body preceding inflammatory joints conditions)		

periodontal-abcess:
hot compress maybe applied to the face until a **dentist** is consulted.

[s]***bergamot**   [s]***chamomile**   [s]***lavender**   [st]***tea-tree**
                                                              - (singularly/
                                                              combined)

abscess-cold:
 [s]***bergamot**   [s]***chamomile**   [s]***lavender**   [st]***tea-tree**.

abscess-warm:
  [**st**] onion;   (onion poultice).

* **Clients general health** should also be considered - advice on a **non-toxic diet** - also **vitamin** and **mineral** supplementation maybe needed, especially if condition is recurrent.

---

acne:
is caused by over-activity of the skins sebaceous glands - combined with bacterial infections - excess sebum poured onto the skin surface where it is mixed with dirt - fluff from clothing - sticks to sebum forming a **breeding ground** for bacteria - pores become blocked - forms blackheads - congested hair follicles become infected - gives rise to blemishes which then seeps out infecting surrounding tissue ~ at puberty, sebaceous glands are under the influence of **androgens** - male / hormones which grow in size increasing production of sebum ~ **testosterone** - appears to be the most potent circulating androgen for sebaceous cell stimulation - **adrenal** - **ovarian** androgens also stimulate sebaceous secretions ~ **basic acne lesions** in order, increasing severity are; **comedones** - **papules** - **pustules** - **cysts** - these predominantly occur in sebaceous follicles - rapidly colonised by bacteria which thrive in lipid-rich sebum - when this occurs - the cyst of connective tissue cells can destroy epidermal cells - hence permanent scarring - a condition called (cystic acne). **Care needs to be taken**, avoid squeezing or scratching these lesions - a synthetic form of vitamin A – a pharmaceutical medicine called - accutane - isotretinoin - is prescribed by the medical fraternity.

precaution:
acne; **must not** be used during **pregnancy**, or those planning to fall pregnant during the course of treatment as major foetal abnormalities have been traced to accutane. This drug may also cause serious side effects in those who are taking accutane.

Aromatherapy:
acne maybe treated successfully without using potentially dangerous drugs or chemicals – plant essences are used externally to clear infection - reduce sebum production - local rub - to stimulate circulation - help body eliminate toxins - recommend **non-toxic** diet - **most important** part of *t*reatment - combined with good hygiene - exercise - medative relaxation - a good night's sleep.

microbes:
a list of specific pure essential plant essences being more effective with specific microbes. (streptococcus – gonococcus – pneumococcus).

[**st**]*tea tree;   (specific to - staphylococcus aurens = ie; infected wounds).

bactericide-essences:
kills bacteria - most pure essential essences are **bactericidal-agents - antiseptic-agents**.

[**st**] swt basil	[s] benzoin	[s]***bergamot**	[s] chamomiles
[**st**]***cajeputi**	[**st**] cinnamon leaf	[**st**] cumin	[**st**]***clove bud**
[s] elemi	[**st**]***garlic**	[s] helichrysum	[**st**]***eucalyptus** radiata
[s] immortelle	[**st**]***juniper berry**	[s]***lavender**	[**n**]***lemon**
[**st**] lemongrass	[**n**] lime	[**st**] litsea cubeba	[**st**]***myrrh** (thyroid)
[s] myrtle	[s]***neroli**	[**st**]***niaouli**	[**st**] origanum
[**st**] palmarosa	[s] rose	[**st**]***rosemary**	[**st**] rosewood
[s]***sandalwood**	[**st**] spruce	[**st**]***tea tree**	[**st**] swt thyme.

abscess-boils:

[s]***sandalwood**;	(specific to – kidney infections).
[**st**]***swt thyme**;	(specific to – e. **coli** - found in some kidney infections).
[n]***lemon**;	(specific to – c. diphtheria).
[**st**]***cinnamon leaf**;	(specific to – typhus bacillus).
[**st**]***clove bud**;	(specific to – m. tuberculosis).

cicatrisant-essences:

[s]***lavender**;	(soothing - healing, promotes new cell growth).

antidepressive-essences:

[s]***bergamot**;	(also **astringent - antidepressant** - as depression exacerbates condition).

sebum-balancer-essences:

[**n**]***geranium**;	(facial massage, crèmes, skin cleansing, toning lotion between treatments).

lymphatic-stimulants:

[s] cypress	[**st**]***rosemary**	[n]***geranium**	[**st**] swt fennel seed
[s] immortelle	[**n**] lemon;	(use in body massage to **stimulate lymphatic system**).	

best-essences:

[s] khellin	[**st**] anise	[**st**] swt basil	[s] bergamot.
[s]***helichrysum**;	> jojoba oil.		

Get Your Health Back with Alternative Medicines

<u>detoxicant-essences</u>:

[**st**]***juniper berry**;	(has a **detoxifying** effect on One's system).
[s] neroli;	(firms and helps the tissues).

[s] immortelle	[s] lavender	[**n**] lemon	[**st**] lemongrass
[**st**] niaouli	[s] patchouli.		

<u>lymph-cleansing-essences</u>:

[**n**] birch bud	[**st**] cajeputi	[**st**] camphor	[s] cedarwood atlas
[s] chamomiles	[**st**] eucalyptus radiata.		

<u>antiseptic-antiviral-essences</u>:

[**st**] palmarosa   [**st**] peppermint.

<u>antibacterial-essences</u>:

[**st**] palmarosa   [**st**] peppermint.

<u>stimulant-essences</u>:   (these essences very stimulating to the mind - do not use at night time).

[**st**] black pepper	[**b**] pettitgrain	[**st**] pine needles	[**st**] rosemary.

<u>sedating-essences</u>:

[s]***sandalwood**;	(mix with other **anti-acne essences**).
[**st**] spearmint;	(undiluted, maybe more effective with **tea tree**).

<u>reduces pus</u>:

[**st**]***tea tree**   [**st**] swt thyme   [s] vetivert.

<u>reduces scarring</u>:

  [s]***lavender**   [s]***neroli**.

<u>medium</u>:

* As **acne** clears - blend **wheatgerm** into **carrier** oil with **lavender** and **neroli** to reduce scarring.
* If **Client** is past mid-twenties - this may be due to an allergy - a different approach is needed.

<u>actinic keratosis</u>:

formation of a hardened growth of tissue - *****artemesia arborescens;** has produced very amazing results.

use **anti-inflammatant-agents - antiallergenic-agents.**

these essences are excellent for abnormal growths - also very sensitive skin - due to its high content of azulene, combined with **1%** solution of **aloe vera gel** works well on severely **damaged cellular tissue.**

<u>anti-inflammatant-essences</u>:

reduces the pain and swelling which accompanies inflammation.

[s]***amyris**	[st]***angelica** root	[s]***bergamot**	[st]***artemesia** arborescens
[n]***calendula**	[s] celery seed	[s]***chamomiles**	[s] clary sage
[st]***eucalyptus** radiata	[s] guaiacwood	[s] helichrysum	[s] immortelle
[s] inula	[s]***khellin**	[s]***lavender**	[s] melissa
[st]***myrrh**	[s] patchouli	[st]***peppermint**	[st] pine needles
[s] rose	[s] sandalwood	[st] santolina	[s] tagetes
[st] yarrow....			
[st]***swt fennel seed**;	(prevents **toxic waste build**-up in body - preceding inflammatory joint conditions).		

antiallergenic-essences:

use these essential essences are used to reduce the effects of **allergens**.

[s] benzoin	[s] bergamot	[n] birch bud	[st] artemesia arborescens
[st] cajeputi	[st] carrot seed	[s] cedarwood atlas	[s]***roman chamomile**
[s] german chamomile	[n] geranium	[b] hyssop	[s] immortelle
[st] juniper berry	[st]**khellin (asthma)	[s] lavender	[s]***melissa**
[st] myrrh	[s] neroli	[st] pine needles	[s]***rose**
[st] rose geranium	[s] sandalwood	[st] tea tree	[st] yarrow.
<u>general</u>:	[s] immortelle	[s] chamomile	[s] melissa
	[st] yarrow.		
<u>skin</u>:	[s] chamomile, german	[s]***melissa**	[s]***rose.**
<u>dry eczema</u>:	[st] rose geranium	[s] sandalwood	[st] tea tree.
<u>weeping eczema</u>:	[st] juniper berry	[s] lavender	[st] myrrh.
<u>sensitive skin</u>:	[st]***artemesia** arborescens; high azulene, effective on eczema, **1%** > **aloe vera** gel.		

---

ageing skin:

pure essential essences which help in the rejuvenation of the skin tissue are called, **rejuvenator-agents**.

<u>rejuvenator-essences</u>:

[s] clary sage	[s] cypress	[s] frankincense	[s] guaiacwood
[n] geranium	[s] helichrysum	[s] jasmine	[n]***lemon**
[s] linden blossom	[eu]***spikenard**	[st] swt thyme.	

for ageing skin – congestive skin – elasticity – wrinkles:

the skin may deteriorate in numerous ways when ageing - for example - discolouration - dryness - a crepey appearance - sagging - thread or surface veins (capillaries) in the cheeks.

Aromatherapy treatments - also incorporating pure essential plant essences made into crèmes - helps minimise all these problems ~ a good supply of oxygen to growing layer of skin is important in maintaining skins health - appearance - massage helps to stimulate the circulation.

<u>face massage</u>:

must always be very gentle, ultra-light to avoid stretching the skin more, but a vigorous scalp massage will increase blood circulation to the whole head, including the face ~ anyone can do this for themselves daily - a face massage should be left to a trained therapist - should form the basis of treatment for the above mentioned problems - the outermost, visible layer of the skin, the **epidermis**, is composed of dead cells, the health - appearance of your skin depends to a large degree on the new layer of cells constantly growing beneath it - **renewal rate** may slow with age, so **cytophylactic essences** (stimulate healthy new growth) are important to counteract this.

<u>neroli-lavender-essences</u>:

are the best essential essences for this - most skins become less oily with age, at its peak during adolescence, this is due to the skins natural lubricant oil called **sebum**, which declines with age, quality and quantity. Use in a blend with either **geranium – jasmine – neroli –** or **rose** will help to restore this natural balance to some degree, will also help to add, **avocado – jojoba – meadowfoam** or **peach kernel** as a **carrier** oil - excellent made into crèmes.

<u>frankincense-essence</u>:

very good on older skin, with those already listed; add **sandalwood - patchouli** - these help to counteract dullness / crepey texture, especially combined with regular massage if in spite of such treatment, skin looks **muddy** in colour, face-paks with **yoghurt** help to give a fresher appearance - simple face-pak made with fresh **avocado pulp** or ground **almonds** mixed with a little **honey** are also very good for older skin.

surface veins:

broken capillaries - are sometimes a problem for older women - **chamomile - rose** - helps to diminish this problem - though it maybe several months before a real improvement is seen.

treatment:

Use in massage blends - crèmes - lotions apply daily - must be done regularly for best effect.

Treatment to continue for some time - best to alternate essences rather than use them all at the same time.

toxins:

Avoid extremes of heat - very hot drinks - smoking - alcohol - your skin reflects the general health of your body - everything contributing to this will delay or minimise ravages time makes on skin - exercise - excellent nutrition - plenty of fresh water - adequate sleep - avoidance of unnecessary pollutants.

wrinkles-rejuvenation:

connective tissue which forms a great part of layers (dermis) of the skin losing its elasticity is why wrinkles form - young skin snaps back to its original state - as skin ages - neglect - it doesn't snap back into shape - stays stretched - like old elastic - poor diet - too much sun - smoking - helps deteriorate the problem - regular massage with plant essences can help in reducing the effects of wrinkles - although the best time to apply such treatment would ideally be - before wrinkles start - massage stimulates local circulation - this ensures a good supply of oxygen to minute blood vessels in the inner layers of the skin - vigorous scalp massages stimulates the whole head - massage - the imput of plenty of oxygen also helps to tone facial muscles underlying the skin - gives a more youthful appearance.

two important essences:

- [s]***frankincense**; (skin **preservative,** may reduce existing wrinkles, helps prevent future wrinkles).
- [s]***neroli**; (**stimulates** the body into making healthy new cells).

essential carrier oils:

these are also very important too - richer oils such as **avocado - jojoba - meadowfoam** oils are best - with addition of 25 % **wheatgerm** oil.

exercise:

also important too - also massage - to increase circulation - to improve muscle tone.

nutrition:

also important especially foods which supply important nutrients such as vitamins B, C, E, plus a good vitamin - mineral supplement.

toxins:

no **smoking - alcohol** - excess **tea** or **coffee** - these substances lower the vitality of One's skin - increasing wrinkles.

essences to use for rejuvenating Ones skin:

- [s] benzoin; (for cracked - dry skin - making it more elastic).
- [**n**] geranium; (helps to restore natural balance).
- [**st**] swt basil; (stimulates sluggish - congested skin).
- [s] jasmine, (carriers **avocado – jojoba** or **peach kernel** oil).
- [s] rose, (carriers **avocado – jojoba** or **peach kernel** oil).
- [s] neroli, (carriers **avocado – jojoba** or **peach kernel** oil).
- [s] rose + [s] neroli; (both for **elasticity** and a little **wheatgerm** made into crèmes also).
- [**st**] carrot seed; (**tone - elasticity** - age spots - wrinkles - due to action on **epidermal** cells).

[s] swt orange;	(good for **collagen** formation).	
[s] celery seed;	(puffiness - redness due to water-logged skin).	
[s] frankincense;	(cytophylactic - tonic to wrinkles to counteracts dullness and crepey texture).	
[s] sandalwood +	[s] patchouli;	(especially when combined in a regular massage).
[s] patchouli;	(**elasticity** - for loose skin due to excessive dieting).	
[s] chamomiles;	(broken capillaries - improving elasticity).	
[s] sandalwood;	(mixed with **cocoa butter** - **elasticity**).	
[s] lavender;	(**cicatrisant** - **cytophylactic** essence use for elasticity).	
[s] neroli;	(**cytophylactic** essence use for **elasticity**).	
[st] rosewood;	(**elasticity**.)	
[s] sandalwood;	(wrinkles etc).	
[s] jasmine;	(**elasticity**.)	
[s] lavender + [s] rose;	(carrier important, **avocado – jojoba** – plus **25** % **wheatgerm** oil.)	
[s] neroli +	[s] mandarin;	(elasticity).
[st] swt fennel seed;	(has a **cleansing** and **tonic** action on the skin for wrinkles).	
all **cytophylactics:**	[st] galbanum;	[st] elemi; [s] violet leaf; [s] rose.

<u>yoghurt face pack</u>:

*gives a fresher appearance - **avocado pulp** or **ground almond** mixed with **honey** - exercise to increase circulation - *improve muscle tone - good diet - plenty foods high in vitamins B, C, E, vitamin and mineral supplements - *No **alcohol + smoking + caffeine** - they lower vitality of skin - tendency to increase wrinkles.

athletes foot:

a superficial fungal infection of the skin of the feet.

antifungal-essences:

[**st**] angelica root	[**n**]***calendula**	[**st**] camphor	[s] cedarwood atlas
[**st**] coriander	[**st**] cinnamon leaf	[**st**] citronella	[s] elemi
[**st**] swt fennel seed	[**st**] garlic	[s]***helichrysum**	[s] hypericum
[s] immortelle	[s] lavender	[**st**] lemongrass	[s] swt marjoram
[**st**]***myrrh**	[**st**] nutmeg	[s] patchouli	[**n**] common sage
[**st**] savory	[s] tagetes	[**st**]***tea tree**	[**st**]***swt thyme**.

---

baldness:

the age, the degree of thinning, also the hair pattern associated with (common baldness, male-pattern baldness) are determined by male hormones called **androgens**, also the hereditary factors. **Androgens** also involved in promoting of normal sexual development, in recent years **minoxidil** (rogaine), **a potent vaso-dilator drug** used to treat high blood pressure, has been applied topically to stimulate hair regrowth in those experiencing thinning hair associated with common-baldness - it will not help those who are bald. As **minoxidil** increases blood flow in the skin, it's believed to stimulate existing hair follicles to become more active. One side effect of **minoxidil** tablets is increasing facials hair (experienced). There are less toxic methods of increasing hair regrowth.

suggested-essences:

here are some pure essential essences which are reputed to stimulate the regrowth of hair.

[**n**]***birch bud**	[s] clary sage	[s] lavender	[**st**] rosemary.

carrier oils:

***jojoba** oil,   organic coconut oil,   macadamia oil,   meadowfoam oil.

reputed blend:

this blend I used for a **Client** worked very well.

[st] swt basil   [n] geranium   [s] ylang-ylang   > **jojoba** oil - **meadowfoam** oil.

medium:

application: (apply small amount all over scalp, massage in - **am / pm** ~ scalp needs to be washed daily.

---

bites:

bites from either,	**bees - wasps - spiders - ants - fleas - lice.**
snakes:	[st]***angelica root**; (neutralises snake bite venom)....
funnel webs:	[s] patchouli [st] tea tree [st]***angelica root**; (neutralises).
bees:	[s]***chamomiles** [s]***lavender** [n]***lemon**.
wasps:	[st]***swt basil**.
insect bites:	[st]***cajeputi** [st]***swt basil**.
repels insects:	[st] clove bud + [s] swt orange + [n] lemon. (excellent)..
fleas-deterrent:	[st] cajeputi; (rub pet with diluted **cajeputi** blend).
lice:	[st] cajeputi [st] tea tree.

blepharitis:

inflammation of the eyelids - use **anti-inflammatant-agents** to reduce inflammation..

anti-inflammatant-essences:

[st]*swt fennel seed	[s] roman chamomile	[s] clary sage	[n]*jojoba
[n] lemon	[n] comfrey root wash	[n] myrtle hydrosyl.	

---

blisters:

a vesicle, or small sac of damaged fluid, due to persistent friction, example shoe rubbing heels etc, pinching or bruising - with **blood blisters**, has a bloody content - maybe caused by a pinch or bruise.

suggested-essences:

[s]*lavender	[st] eucalyptus radiata.

---

boils - carbuncles:

hard, round, deep painful inflammations of subcutaneous tissue which cause necrosis (death) - pus formation (pus).

resolvent-essences:

dissolves boils - swellings.

[st] swt fennel seed	[st] galbanum	[st] garlic	[st] grapefruit
[b] hyssop	[st] rosemary.		

anti-inflammatant-essences:

reduces the pain and swelling which accompanies inflammation.

[s]***amyris**	[st]***angelica root**	[s]***bergamot**	[st]***artemesia** arborescens
[n]***calendula**	[st]***cedarwood atlas**	[s] celery seed	[s]***chamomiles**
[s] clary sage	[s]***eucalyptus radiata**	[st]***swt fennel seed**	[s] guaiacwood
[s] helichrysum	[s] immortelle	[s] inula	[s]***khellin**
[s]***lavender**	[st]***myrrh**	[s] patchouli	[st]***peppermint**
[st] pine needles	[s] rose	[s] sandalwood	[**st**] santolina
[s] tagetes	[st] turmeric	[**st**] yarrow.	

---

bruising:

discolouring of skin due to trauma.

suggested-essences:

| [st]***bay laurel** | [st]***black pepper** | [s]***brahami** | [s]***hypericum**. |

---

burns:

Tissue maybe damaged by thermal, electrical, radio-active, or chemical agents, all of which can destroy, **denature**, the **proteins** in the exposed cells and cause cell or death. Such damage is called a burn.

Burns may **disrupt homeostasis** because they destroy the protection afforded by the skin, this creates microbial invasion & infection - loss of fluid - loss of temperature control.

Generally systemic effects of a burn are a greater threat to life than the local effects.

Large **loss of water - plasma - proteins** which cause **shock**.

Bacterial infection.

Reduced circulation of blood.

Reduced production of urine.

classification:

A **first-degree burn** involves only the surface epidermis.

characterised by; Mild pain, erythema (**redness**) - dry skin - slight oedema - no blisters.

It will usually heal within a couple of days, accompanied by flaky or peeling skin.

A typical sunburn is a good example of a first-degree burn.

classification:

A **second-degree burn** involves the **entire epidermis**, or varying portions of the dermis - skin function is lost. In a **superficial, second-degree burn** - the deeper layers of the epidermis are injured.

characterised by; pain - redness - blister formation - as well as marked oedema.

This will probably heal within 7-10 days with only minor scarring.

In a **deep second-degree burn**, theres destruction of the epidermis as well as the upper level of the dermis.

The epidermal derivatives, such as hair follicles, sebaceous glands, and sweat glands are not usually damaged.

If there is no infection, **deep second-degree burns** heal without grafting about **3 - 4** weeks.

Scarring may result.

First and **Second-degree burns** are collectively referred to as **partial-thickness** burns.

classification:

A **third-degree burn** or **full-thickness burn** involves destruction of the epidermis - dermis - epidermal derivatives - the skin functions are lost.

characterised by; Such burns vary in experience from **marble** to **mahogany** coloured, to charred, dry wounds. There is marked **oedema**, and such a burn is not usually painful to touch due to the destruction of nerve endings. Regeneration is slow, and much **granulation tissue** forms before being covered by epithelium.

Even if **skin-grafting** has been quickly started, **third-degree burns** rapidly contract and produce scarring.

Aromatherapy:

Treatment for **first** and **second-degree burns** is; submerge affected area into a **lavender** solution to cover the burnt area completely, until the pain has subsided.

This will remove the pain from the burn, and aid in quick healing, leaving **minimal scarring**.

May take up to **20** minutes depending on the severity of burn.

A1 best essence:

[s]****lavender**; (submerse burnt area into pure undiluted lavender until pain subsides - when pain has subsided there will be no scarring if followed accordingly, approx **20** minutes).

<u>effective-essences:</u>

[s] chamomile	[n] geranium	[s]***helichry-sum**	[s]****lavender**
[st] niaouli	[s] neroli	[st] tea tree.	
<u>carrier oils:</u>	*aloe vera,	calendula oil,	evening primrose oil,	*artemesia arbor.

---

callus:

a hardened and thickened area of skin that is usually seen in the palms of hands - the soles of the feet due to prolonged pressure and friction.

suggested-essences:

[st] clove bud   [st] garlic   [s] swt orange.

---

cellular tissue damage:

damaged cellular tissue - hard to heal skin conditions.

<u>cytophylactic-essences:</u>

which have a therapeutic action when used to regenerate a healthy skin.

[st]***artemesia**	[st]***carrot seed**	[s] clary sage	[s]***frankencense**
[n] geranium	[s]***helichrysum**	[s] immortelle	[s]***lavender**
[s] mandarin	[s]***neroli**	[s]****sweet orange**	[st]***palmarosa**
[s] patchouli	[s]***rose**	[st] rose geranium	[eu] spikenard
[s] tagetes	[s]***tangerine**	[st]***tea tree.**	

chicken pox:

a highly contagious dis-ease which initiates in the respiratory system, caused by the **varicella- zoster virus**.

characterised by; vesicular eruptions on the skin that fill with pus, to form a scab before healing.

Also called varicella [var'-i-SEL-a] (shingles is caused by the latent chicken pox virus)

antipruritic-essences:

using **antipruritic** essences to relieve the severe itching.

[s]***chamomiles**	[s] inula	[s] lavender	[n]***lemon**
[st] peppermint	[st] pine needles	[st]***spearmint**	[st]***tea tree**
[rub] terebinth.			
[st] peppermint +	[st] spearmint;	(makes an excellent cold blend).	

antiviral-essences:

antiviral-agents are used to kill viral organisms.

[st] artemesia/ annua	[s]***bergamot**	[s] elemi	[st]***garlic**
[st] eucalyptus radiata	[n] geranium	[s] helichrysum	[s] immortelle
[s] lavender	[st] spike lavender	[n] lemon	[n] lime
[s] melissa	[st] origanum	[st] palmarosa	[s] rose bulgarian
[st]***tea tree**	[st] swt thyme.		

<u>best antiviral-essences</u>:

[s]***bergamot**;	(is a very powerful **antiviral essence**).
[**st**]***tea tree**;	(very powerful, well known stimulant for **immune response** to infection).
[**st**] eucalyptus radiata;	(is not as powerful as **tea tree**)
<u>mediums</u>:	**bath.**
<u>bath</u>:	(**eucalyptus - chamomile - lavender** in a bath will reduce a fever and ease itching).

---

chilblains:

a recurrent localised itching - swelling - and painful erythema on the fingers - toes - and ears - produced

by mild frostbite - use **cytophylactics - cicatrisants**.

<u>cytophylactic-essences</u>:

helps in the regeneration of new tissue cells,

[**st**]***carrot seed**   [s] chamomile   [s]***frankencense**   [**n**] geranium
[**st**] rose geranium

<u>cicatrisant-essences</u>:

[s]* **benzoin tinctu**re   [s] bergamot   [s] german chamomile   [s] cypress

[s] frankencense   [**n**] geranium   [**n**] lemon   [**st**] rose geranium

<u>carrier oils</u>:

vitamin A – vitamin E – meadowfoam – rosehip seed – sesame seed – wheatgerm oils.

---

cold sores:

A lesion, usually in the oral mucous membrane, caused by **type-1 herpes simplex virus** [HSV], transmitted by oral or respiratory routes. Triggering factors; UV **radiation - hormonal changes - emotional stress - fever blisters**.

antiviral-essences:

Use **antiviral-agents** which kill viral organisms.

[st] artemesia annua	[s]***bergamot**	[s] elemi	[st]***garlic**
[st] eucalyptus radiata	[n] geranium	[s] helichrysum	[s] immortelle
[s] lavender	[st] spike lavender	[n] lemon	[n] lime
[s] melissa	[st] origanum	[st] palmarosa	[s] rose bulgarian
[st]***tea tree**	[st] sweet thyme.		

best antiviral-essences:

[s]***bergamot**; (is a very powerful antiviral essence).

[st]***tea tree**; (very powerful, well known stimulant for immune response to infection).

[st] eucalyptus; (is not as powerful as **tea tree**)

mediums: **bath - vapour - inhalants - these are the best forms of treatments.**

steam inhalant: (steam inhalants best medium, due to fever usually accompanies cold, influenza etc.

massage: (massage is contra-indicated with fever.

vapouriser: (burner - electrical fragrancer - diffusor - simply means of a few drops of essence on light globe. It not only helps the **Client**, but it's one of the best ways to reduce air-borne transmission of infection to other members of their family).

comedo: (black heads or whiteheads)

A collection of sebaceous material /dead cells in hair follicle, excretory duct of sebaceous gland - usually found on **face - chest - back** - occurs mostly during adolescence - called **blackheads** or **whiteheads**.

antiseptic-essences:

helps in **preventing tissue degeneration** - all essential essences **inhibit** the growth of organisms bacteria / germs, some essences being more effective than others, indicated by * also in the controlling of infections.

[s] amyris	[st] bay laurel	[s] benzoin	[s]*__bergamot__
[n] birch bud	[st] black pepper	[st] cajeputi	[st] caraway seed
[s] cedarwood atlas	[s] german chamomile	[s] roman chamomile	[st] cinnamon leaf
[s] clary sage	[st] clove bud	[st] cumin	[s] cypress
[st]*__eucalyptus__ radiata	[st] swt fennel seed	[s] fir needle	[s]*__frankincense__
[n] geranium	[st] ginger	[st] grapefruit	[s]*__helichrysum__
[b] hyssop	[s] jasmine	[st]*__juniper berry__	[st] lavandin
[s]*__lavender__	[st] spike lavender	[n] lemon	[s] lemongrass
[n] lime	[s] sweet marjoram	[st] may chang	[st] myrrh (thyroid)
[n] myrtle	[st] niaouli	[st] nutmeg	[s] swt orange
[st] origanum	[st] palmarosa	[s] parsley herb	[s] patchouli
[st]*__peppermint__	[st] pine needles	[s] rose	[st] rose geranium
[st]*__rosemary__	[s] rosewood	[s]*__sandalwood__	[st] spikenard
[s] tagetes	[s] tangerine	[st]*__tea tree__	[st] swt thyme
[s] verbena, lemon	[s] vetivert	[s] violet leaf	[st] yarrow
[s] ylang-ylang...			

excretory-antiseptic: [st]*__juniper berry__.

conjunctivitis:

Infections of the eyes.

suggested-essences:

[s] clary sage [s] lavender [s] rose [s] roman chamomile

[st] swt fennel seed.

---

corns:

are a painful conical thickening of the skin found principally over toe joints and between the toes it maybe soft or hard, depending on the location - hard corns are usually found over the toe joints, and soft corns are usually found between the fourth and fifth toes.

cytophylactic-essences:

cellular regenerators - helps in the formation of new tissue cells.

[st]*artemesia	[st]*carrot seed	[s] clary sage	[s]*frankencense
[n] geranium	[s]*helichrysum	[s] immortelle	[s]*lavender
[s] mandarin	[s]*neroli	[s]*swt orange	[st]*palmarosa
[s] patchouli	[s]*rose	[st] rose geranium	[s] spikenard
[s] tagetes	[s]*tangerine	[st]*tea tree.	

emollient-essences:

are soothing and softening to the skin.

| [s] cedarwood atlas | [s] chamomiles | [n] geranium | [n] helichrysum |
| [b] hyssop | [s] immortelle | [s] jasmine | [s] lavender |

[n] lemon	[s] linden blossom	[s] mandarin	[s] neroli
[s] rose	[s] sandalwood	[s] tagetes	[s] tangerine
[s] verbena, lemon.			

carrier oils:

vitamin A oil - **vitamin** E oil - **rosehip seed** oil - **sesame seed** oil - **meadowfoam** oil - **wheatgerm** oil.

---

dandruff:

a condition of dry skin of the scalp ie; - toxic chemicals in **shampoo - emotional - dietary**.

suggested-essences:

[st] swt basil	[s] cedarwood atlas	[s] clary sage	[n] geranium
[st] juniper berry	[s]***lavender** (tonic)	[st] rosemary.	

---

decubitus ulcers:

are commonly known as bedsores or pressure sores which are caused by a chronic deficiency of blood to the tissues which have been subjected to prolonged pressure of the overlying bony projection against objects, ie; beds -casts - splints - resulting in tissue ulceration - where small breaks in **epidermis** become infected. Sensitive subcutaneous and deeper tissues are then damaged. These ulcers most frequently are seen in bed-ridden patients confined over long periods. Most common sites are; **buttocks - sacrum - heels - ankles** - skin over other large bony projections - main cause for pressure is from infrequent turning to alternate positioning - malnutrition - trauma - maceration of skin - maceration only occurs from being left in urine - faeces - or perspiration soaked bedding.

Use **anti-inflammatants - cicatrisants - cytophylactics - rejuvenators - rubefacients**.

<u>anti-inflammatant-essences</u>:

reduces **pain** and **swelling** of **inflammation**.

[s]***ammi visnaga**	[s]***amyris**	[st]***angelica root**	[st]***artemesia** arborescens
[s]***bergamot**	[n]***calendula**	[st]***cedarwood atlas**	[s] celery seed
[s]***chamomiles**	[s] clary sage	[st]***eucalyptus** radiata	[st] swt fennel seed
[s] guaiacwood	[s] helichrysum	[s] immortelle	[s] inula
[s]***lavender**	[st]***myrrh**	[s] patchouli	[st]***peppermint**
[st] pine needles	[s] rose	[s] sandalwood	[st] santolina
[s] tagetes	[st] turmeric	[st] yarrow.	

<u>cicatrisant-essences</u>:

helps with the **formation** of **scar tissue**.

[s] bergamot	[st] cajeputi	[s] chamomiles	[st] clove bud
[s] cypress	[st] eucalyptus radiata	[s] frankencense	[st] garlic
[n] geranium	[s] hypericum	[b] hyssop	[s] jasmine
[st] juniper berry	[st] lavandin	[s] lavender	[n] lemon
[st] niaouli	[s] patchouli	[st] rose geranium	[st] rosemary
[n] common sage	[st] tea tree	[rub] terebinth	[st] swt thyme
[st] yarrow.	[st]***artemesia** arborescens; (amazing results - **actinic keratosis**)		

<u>cytophylactic-essences</u>:

helps in the **formation** of **new tissue cells**.

[**st**]***artemesia** arbores	[**st**]***carrot seed**	[s] clary sage	[s]***frankencense**
[**n**] geranium	[s]***helichrysum**	[s] immortelle	[s]***lavender**
[s] mandarin	[s]***neroli**	[s]***swt orange**	[**st**]***palmarosa**
[s] patchouli	[s]***rose**	[**st**] rose geranium	[s] spikenard
[s] tagetes	[s]***tangerine**	[**st**]***tea tree**.	

<u>rejuvenator-essences</u>:

rejuvenator-essences help in the **rejuvenation** of the **skin tissue**.

[s] benzoin	[**s**]***carrot seed**	[s] frankencense	[s] jasmine
[s] lavender	[**n**] lemon	[**st**] myrrh	[s] neroli
[s] patchouli	[**st**] peppermint	[**b**] pettitgrain	[s] rose
[**st**] rosemary	[s] sandalwood.		

<u>rubefacient-essences</u>:

rubefacient-essences create warmth to the skin by increasing the blood flow to the area.

[**st**]***black pepper**	[**st**] camphor	[**st**]***ginger**	[**st**]***eucalyptus** radiata
[**st**]***juniper berry**	[s] swt marjoram	[**st**] origanum	[**st**] pimento
[**st**] pine needles	[**st**]***rosemary**	[**rub**] terebinth.	

lupus - bedsores:

[s]***benzoin** [**st**] clove bud [s] frankencense

<u>scar tissue</u>:

[**st**] myrrh [s] patchouli.

---

eczema:

is an acute - chronic superficial skin inflammation - <u>characterised</u> by; **itching - swelling - blistering - redness - oozing - crusting - scaly skin** - due to **stress** or **chronic dermatitis** -

use **antiallergen-agents - anti-inflammatant-agents**.

<u>antiallergenic-essences</u>:

use these **antiallergenic-essences** to reduce the effects of **allergens**.

[s] benzoin	[s] bergamot	[**n**] birch bud	[**st**] cajeputi
[**st**] carrot seed	[s] cedarwood atlas	[s]***chamo-miles**	[**n**] geranium
[**b**] hyssop	[**st**] pine needles	[s] neroli	[**st** tea tree.

<u>general</u>:	[s] immortelle	[s] chamomile	[s] melissa	[**st**] yarrow.
<u>skin</u>:	[**st**] artemesia arbores	[s] german chamomile	[s] melissa	[s] rose.
<u>sensitive skin</u>:	[**st**]***arteme-sia** arb;	(high azulene - effective eczema, **1**% sol > **aloe vera** gel).		
<u>dry eczema</u>:	[**st**] rose geranium	[s] sandalwood	[**st**] tea tree.	
<u>weeping eczema</u>:	[**st**] juniper berry	[s] lavender	[**st**] myrrh.	

<u>anti-inflammatant-essences</u>:

reduces **pain** and **swelling** of inflammation.

[s]***ammi visnaga**	[s]***amyris**	[st]***angelica root**	[st]***artemesia** arborescens
[s]***bergamot**	[n]***calendula**	[st]***cedarwood atlas**	[s] celery seed
[s]***chamomiles**	[s] clary sage	[st]***eucalyptus** radiata	[st]***swt fennel seed**
[s] guaiacwood	[s] helichrysum	[s] immortelle	[s] inula
[s]***lavender**	[st]***myrrh**	[s] patchouli	[st]***peppermint**
[st] pine needles	[s] rose	[s] sandalwood	[st] santolina
[s] tagetes	[st] turmeric	[st] yarrow.	

<u>elasticity ~ skin</u>:

pure essential plant essences which are beneficial in helping to retain the **skins elasticity**.

<u>elasticity-essences</u>:

[st] sweet basil	[s] benzoin	[st] carrot seed	[s] chamomiles
[s] frankencense	[s]***jasmine**	[s]***lavender**	[st] lemongrass
[s] linden blossom	[s]***mandarin**	[st] myrrh	[s] neroli
[s] rose.			

<u>best combination</u>:	[s]***jasmine**	[s]***mandarin**	[s]***lavender**.
<u>returns skin colour</u>:	[s]***tangerine**.		
<u>dry-mature-ageing-skin</u>:	[s] vetivert.		
<u>puffiness</u>:	[s] celery seed	[st] swt fennel seed.	

<u>wrinkles:</u>

[**st**] carrot seed	[s] clary sage	[**st**] swt fennel seed	[s] frankencense
[**n**] geranium	[s] guaiacwood	[s] helichrysum	[s] jasmine
[**n**] lemon	[s] palmarosa	[s] patchouli	[s] rose
[**st**] rose geranium	[**st**] rosewood	[s] sandalwood	[s] spikenard
[s] tangerine	[s] vetivert	[s] ylang-ylang.	

<u>carrier oils:</u>

vitamin A - **vitamin** E - **rosehip** - **sesame seed** - **jojoba** - **wheatgerm** oils.

---

elephantiasis:

long-standing oedema of one or both lower extremities - sometimes of the arms or other body parts - which is due to **lymphatic obstruction** - the limb may become tremendously swollen and hardened - the skin surface may resemble an elephants leg - **elephantiasis** maybe due to **filariasis**, a parasitic infestation - also causes **congestive heart failure** and **chronic obstruction** of the **lymphatic vessels**.

<u>suggested-essence:</u>

[s] brahmi.

---

erythema:

is redness of the skin caused by engorgement of capillaries in the lower layers of the skin - **erythema** occurs with any **skin injury - infection - inflammation** - use **anti-inflammatant-agents**.

<u>anti-inflammatant-agents</u>:

reduces the **pain** and **swelling** of inflammation.

[s]***ammi visnaga**	[s]***amyris**	[s]***angelica root**	[s]***artemesia** arborescens
[s]***bergamot**	[n]***calendula**	[s]***cedarwood atlas**	[s] celery seed
[s]***chamomiles**	[s] clary sage	[st]***eucalyptus radiata**	[s] guaiacwood
[s] helichrysum	[s] immortelle	[s] inula	[s]***lavender**
[s]***myrrh**	[s] patchouli	[st]***peppermint**	[st] pine needles
[s] rose	[s] sandalwood	[st] santolina	[s] tagetes
[st] turmeric	[st] yarrow		

[st]***swt fennel seed**; (prevents **toxic waste build-up** in body preceding inflammatory joint conditions).

---

german measles:

Is a highly contagious Dis-ease that initiates in respiratory system - it is caused by the **rubella virus** - characterised by a rash of small red spots on the skin. Also called **rubella** - **viruses** are **invading agents** responsible for most **epidemic illnesses** - including **influenza - chicken pox - small pox - poliomyelitis - measles - colds** - also a great many vague undiagnosed fevers - many instances of **diarrhoea** are due to **viral infections.**

Some forms of **pneumonia** originate from **viral** infections - while others are of **bacterial** in origin.

Use **antiviral-essences - antipruritic-essences.**

antiviral-agents:

use **antiviral** agents which kill viral organisms.

[**st**] artemesia annua	[s]***bergamot**	[s] elemi	[**st**]***garlic**
[**n**] geranium	[s] helichrysum	[s] immortelle	[**st**]***eucalyptus** radiata
[s] lavender	[**st**] spike lavender	[**n**] lemon	[**n**] lime
[s] melissa	[**st**] origanum	[**st**] palmarosa	[s] rose bulgarian
[**st**]***tea tree**	[**st**] swt thyme.		

best antiviral-essences:

[s]***bergamot**;	(is a very powerful **antiviral** essence).
[**st**]***tea tree**;	(very powerful, well known stimulant for immune response to infection).
[**st**] eucalyptus radiata;	(is **not as** powerful as **tea tree**)

antipruritic-essences:

using **antipruritic-essences** to relieve the **severe itching**.

[**st**] swt basil	[s]***bergamot**	[s]***chamomiles**	[**st**]***ginger**
[s] inula	[s] lavender	[**n**]***lemon**	[**st**]***peppermint**
[**st**] pine needles	[**st**]***spearmint**	[**st**]***tea tree**	[rub] terebinth.
[**st**] **peppermint**+	[**st**] **spearmint**;	(makes an excellent cold blend).	

mediums:	**bath - vapour - inhalants** - these are the best forms of treatments for viruses).
bath:	(add a few drops to running bath water, prior to emerging, make sure mixed well).
steam inhalant:	(best medium, due to fever usually accompanying a cold, influenza etc).
massage:	(massage is contra-indicated with fever).

inhale: (maybe inhaled off a tissue or handkerchief,
vapouriser: (whether burner, electrical fragrancer, diffusor - only helps **Client**, one of the best ways of reducing air-borne transmission of infection to their family).

---

herpes:

is any inflammatory skin dis-ease, characterised by the formation of small vesicles in clusters.

it is now usually restricted to such dis-eases caused by **herpes viruses -- herpes simplex** or **herpes zoster**.

go to shingles for more in depth details.

antiviral-essences:

use diluted for herpes or shingles.

[**st**]***swt basil**	[**st**] artemesia annua	[s]***bergamot**	[s] elemi
[**st**]***garlic**	[**st**]***eucalyptus** radiata	[**n**] geranium	[s] helichrysum
[s] lavender	[**st**] spike lavender	[**n**] lemon	[**n**] lime
[s] melissa	[**st**] origanum	[**st**] palmarosa	[s] rose bulgarian
[**st**]***tea tree**	[**st**] swt thyme.		

best essences:

[**st**]***swt basil**;	(use diluted for herpes and shingles).
[s]***bergamot**;	(is a very powerful **antiviral** essence).
[**st**]***tea-tree**;	(very powerful antiviral, known for stimulating body's **immune response** to infection).
[**st**]***eucalyptus** radiata;	(is not quite as powerful as **tea-tree**.)

hives:

an allergic condition presenting on the skin - characterised by elevated patches which are often red and vey itchy - most commonly caused by allergic reactions to specific substances ie; certain **foods additives - medications - physical trauma - emotional stress - chemical reactions** ranging from **food stuffs - bathroom chemicals - dyes - detergents - chloride - fluoride** in town water **supply - infections - physical traumas - flowers - pollen etc** - the list is endless - also called **urticaria**.

Suggested essences to use are **antiallergenic-agents - antipruritic-agents - anti-inflammatant-agents**.

antiallergenic-essences:

use these **antiallergenic-essences** to reduce the effects of **allergens**.

[s] benzoin	[s] bergamot	[n] birch bud	[st] artemesia arborescens
[st] cajeputi	[st] carrot seed	[s] cedarwood atlas	[s]***roman chamomile**
[s] german chamomile	[n] geranium	[b] hyssop	[s] immortelle
[st] juniper berry	[st]**khellin**	[s] lavender	[s]***melissa**
[st] myrrh	[s] neroli	[st] pine needles	[s]***rose**
[st] rose geranium	[s] sandalwood	[st] tea tree	[st] yarrow.

asthma:	[st]**khellin**.			
general:	[s] immortelle	[s] chamomile	[s] melissa	[st] yarrow.
skin:	[s] german chamomile	[st] artemesia arbores.	[s]***melissa**	[s]***rose**.
dry eczema:	[st] rose geranium	[s] sandalwood	[st] tea tree.	

<u>weeping</u> [**st**] juniper [s] lavender [**st**] myrrh.
<u>eczema:</u> berry

<u>sensitive skin</u>**:** [**st**]*artemesia**;** contains **high azulene**, highly effective eczema **1%** > **aloe vera** gel.

<u>antipruritic-
essences</u>**:**

using **antipruritic** essences to relieve the **severe itching**.

[**st**] sweet basil	[s]***bergamot**	[s]***chamomiles**	[**st**]*****ginger**
[s] inula	[s] lavender	[**n**]*****lemon**	[**st**]*****peppermint**
[**st**] pine needles	[**st**]*****spearmint**	[**st**]*****tea tree**	[**rub**] terebinth.
[**st**] **peppermint** +	[**st**] **spearmint;**	(makes an excellent cold blend).	

<u>anti-inflammatant-essences</u>**:**

reduces the **pain** and **swelling** of inflammation.

[s]*****ammi visnaga**	[s]*****amyris**	[**st**]*****angelica root**	[st]*****artemesia** arborescens
[s]*****bergamot**	[**n**]*****calendula**	[**st**]*****cedarwood atlas**	[s] celery seed
[s]*****chamomiles**	[s] clary sage	[**st**]*****eucalyptus radiata**	[s] guaiacwood
[s] helichrysum	[s] immortelle	[s] inula	[s]*****lavender**
[**st**]*****myrrh**	[s] patchouli	[**st**]*****peppermint**	[**st**] pine needles
[s] rose	[s] sandalwood	[**st**] santolina	[s] tagetes
[**st**] turmeric	[**st**] yarrow.		
[**st**]*****swt fennel seed;**	(prevents **toxic waste** build-up)		

impetigo:

superficial skin infection caused by **staphylococci** or **streptococci** most common with children - **Aromatherapists** will not deal with these Dis-eases, but this list shows the plant essences effectiveness in fighting - strengthening the immune system against infectious dis-eases by attacking microbes.

bactericide-essences:

kills bacteria - most pure essential plant essences are **bactericidal-agents - antiseptic-agents.**

[**st**] swt basil	[s] benzoin	[s]***bergamot**	[s] chamomiles
[**st**]***cajeputi**	[**st**] cinnamon leaf	[**st**] cumin	[**st**]***clove** bud
[**st**]***garlic**	[s] elemi	[s] helichrysum	[**st**]***eucalyptus** radiata
[s] immortelle	[**st**]***juniper** berry	[s]***lavender**	[**n**]***lemon**
[**st**] lemongrass	[**n**] lime	[**st**] litsea cubeba	[**st**]***myrrh** (**thyroid**)
[s] myrtle	[s]***neroli**	[**st**]***niaouli**	[**st**] origanum
[**st**] palmarosa	[s] rose	[**st**]***rosemary**	[**st**] rosewood
[s]***sandalwood**	[**st**] spruce	[**st**]***tea tree**	[**st**] swt thyme.

<u>specific / microbes:</u> (staphylococcus – streptococcus – gonococcus – pneumococcus).

<u>specific / microbes:</u> (staphylococcus aurens, ie; infected wounds – abcess – boils).

<u>specific / essences:</u> [**st**] **tea tree.**

<u>specific / microbes:</u> (streptococcus – gonococcus – pneumococcus).

<u>specific / essences:</u>

[s]***sandalwood**; (- specific to - kidney infections)

[st]*swt thyme;	(- specific to - E. coli, found in some **kidney infections**).
[n] lemon;	(- specific to - C. diphtheria).
[st] cinnamon leaf;	(- specific to - typhus bacillus).
[st] clove bud;	(- specific to - M. tuberculosis).

<u>induction</u>:

eases labour pain.

<u>suggested-essences</u>:

[s] clary sage	[s] jasmine	[s] lavender
[st] **pennyroyal**;	**(is known to be fatal ~ do not use at all during pregnancy)**.	

---

insect bites:

using these essences are valuable in **detoxifying** the **circulatory system** of toxic venoms etc.

<u>antivenomous-essences</u>:

antivenoms neutralises poisons.

<u>snake bites</u>:

[st]***angelica root**;	(use neat to wound).
[st] aniseed	
[s]***patchouli**	
[st]***tea tree**	
[st]*swt thyme	
[st]***swt fennel seed**;	(helps in removing toxic poisons from the circulatory system).

suggested-essences:

[st]*angelica root	[st] swt basil	[st] cajeputi	[st] cinnamon leaf
[st]*swt fennel seed	[st] parsley herb	[s]*patchouli	[st] peppermint
[st] spearmint	[st] yarrow.		

antidote to insect bites:

[st] cajeputi

anti-inflammatant-essences:

reduces the **pain** and **swelling** of inflammation.

[st]*angelica root	[s]*bergamot	[n]*calendula	[st]*eucalyptus radiata
[s]*lavender	[st]*myrrh	[s] patchouli	[st]*peppermint
[st] pine needles	[s] tagetes	[st] yarrow.	

antimicrobial-essences:

[st] myrrh	[eu] spikenard	[s] tagetes	[st]*swt thyme.

antitoxin-detoxify-circulatory system:

[st]*angelica root;	(stimulates the circulation, to rid the body and brain of toxins).
[s]*neroli;	(for local circulation)
[st]*niaouli;	(for local circulation)

[st] aniseed	[st]*swt basil	[st] black pepper	[n] birch bud

[st]*swt fennel seed	[s] frankencense	[st]*garlic	[st]*juniper berry
[s] lavender	[n]*lemon	[st]*swt thyme.	[st]*yarrow.

---

odours:

to eliminate unwanted or unpleasant odours.

[st] cardamom;   (uplifting incense - cigarette smoke and others).

<u>deodourant-essences</u>:

destroys the **bacteria** causing the odour.

[s] benzoin	[s]*bergamot	[st] citronella	[s]*clary sage
[st] coriander	[s]*cypress	[n] geranium	[st]*eucalyptus radiata
[s]*lavender	[st] lemongrass	[st] myrrh	[s]*neroli
[s] patchouli	[b]*pettitgrain	[st] pine needles	[st]*rose geranium
[st]*rosewood...			

---

papule:

is a small round skin elevation varying in size from a pinpoint to that of a split pea - one example, a pimple.

<u>antiseptic-essences</u>:

helps in the **prevention** of **tissue degeneration** - also in the controlling of infections.

[s] amyris	[st] bay laurel	[s] benzoin	[s]*bergamot
[n] birch bud	[st] black pepper	[st] cajeputi	[st] caraway seed

[s] cedarwood atlas	[s] german chamomile	[s] roman chamomile	[st] cinnamon leaf
[s] clary sage	[st] clove bud	[st] cumin	[s] cypress
[st]***eucalyptus** radiata	[st] swt fennel seed	[s] fir needle	[s]***frankincense**
[n] geranium	[st] ginger	[st] grapefruit	[s]***helichrysum**
[b] hyssop	[s] jasmine	[st]***juniper berry**	[st] lavandin
[s]***lavender**	[st] spike lavender	[n] lemon	[st] lemongrass
[n] lime	[s] sweet marjoram	[st] may chang	[st] myrrh (thyroid)
[n] myrtle	[st] niaouli	[st] nutmeg	[s] sweet orange
[st] origanum	[st] palmarosa	[s] parsley herb	[s] patchouli
[st]***peppermint**	[st] pine needles	[s] rose	[st] rose geranium
[st]***rosemary**	[s] rosewood	[s]***sandalwood**	[st] spikenard
[s] tagetes	[s] tangerine	[st]***tea tree**	[st] swt thyme
[s] verbena, lemon	[s] vetivert	[s] violet leaf	[st] yarrow
[s] ylang-ylang.	jojoba oil….		

<u>excretory-antiseptic:</u> [st]***juniper berry.**

---

pediculosis: (head-lice)

is an infestation of lice - blood-feeding ectoparasitic insects of the order Phthiraptera. The condition can occur in almost any species of warm-blooded animal (i.e., mammals - birds), including humans - though **pediculosis,** in humans may properly refer to **lice** infestation of any part of the body, the term is sometimes used loosely to refer to **pediculosis capitis**, the infestation of the human head with the specific head louse - for treatment of head lice and further infesting use **pediculosis essences.**

parasiticide-essences:

rids scabies - lice - fleas - a diluted parasitic blend - local application.

[st] aniseed	[st] caraway	[st] cinnamon leaf	[st] citronella
[st] clove bud	[st] cumin	[st]***eucalyptus** radiata	[st] garlic
[s] lavender	[n] lemon	[st] lemongrass	[n] myrtle
[st] origanum	[st] peppermint	[st] rose geranium	[st] rosemary
[st] tea tree	[st] swt thyme.		
[st] citronella;	(this is a good blend > **coconut** oil - rub into scalp - leave over-night - washout - use for weekly preventative during head lice season).		
<u>diluted application</u>:	[st] cinnamon leaf.		
<u>head-pubic-lice</u>:	[st] cajeputi.		
<u>repels fleas - lice</u>:	[st]***eucalyptus**	[n] geranium	[s] lavender	[n] lemon
	[st]***pennyroyal**	[st]***rosemary**	[st]*tea tree.	

---

perspiration:

is the substance which is produced by the **sudoriferous** glands which contains; **water - salts - urea - uric acid - amino acids - ammonia - sugar - lactic acid - ascorbic acid -** maintains body temperature - eliminates wastes.

sudorific-essences:

use **sudorific-agents** to induce sweating.

[st] angelica root	[st]*swt basil	[st] bay laurel	[st] cajeputi
[st] camphor	[st] cardamom	[s]*chamomile	[st] cinnamon leaf
[s] dill	[st] swt fennel seed	[s] frankencense	[st] garlic
[st] ginger	[b] hyssop	[st]*juniper berry	[s] lavender
[s] linden blossom	[s] melissa	[st] myrrh	[st] origanum
[st]*peppermint	[st] pine needles	[st]*rosemary	[st]*tea tree.

antisudorific-essences:

use **antisudorific-agents** to reduce sweating.

[s] clary sage	[st] cypress	[s] elemi	[n] common sage.

---

phlebitis:

inflammation of a peripheral vein, particularly of the lower extremities.

use **anti-inflammatant-agents** to reduce pain and swellings of inflammation.

anti-inflammatant-essences:

reduces the **pain** and **swelling** of inflammation.

[s]*ammi visnaga	[s]*amyris	[st]*angelica root	[st]*artemesia arborescens
[s]*bergamot	[n]*calendula	[st]*cedarwood atlas	[s] celery seed

[s]***chamomiles**	[s] clary sage	[st]***eucalyptus** radiata	[s] guaiacwood
[s] helichrysum	[s] immortelle	[s] inula	[s]***lavender**
[st]***myrrh**	[s] patchouli	[st]***peppermint**	[st] pine needles
[s] rose	[s] sandalwood	[st] santolina	[s] tagetes
[st] turmeric	[st] yarrow.		
[st]***swt fennel seed**;	(helps prevent **toxic waste build-up** body preceding inflammatory joint conditions).		

---

pruritis:

is severe itching, one of the most common of dermalogical disorders.

use **antipruritic-agents** to relieve severe itching.

<u>antipruritic-essences</u>:

[s] bergamot	[st]***black pepper**	[st] carrot seed	[s]***chamomile**
[s] clary sage	[s] inula	[s] lavender	[n]***lemon**
[s] patchouli	[st]***peppermint**	[st]***pine needles**	[st]***spearmint**
[st] tea tree	[rub] terebinth.		

<u>infections</u>:	maybe caused by skin disorders.
<u>cancer-kidney-failure</u>:	systemic disorders.
<u>emotional stress</u>:	psychogenic factors or [ayurveda] **pitta doshas** are out of balance.
<u>excellent cold blend is</u>;	**peppermint + spearmint**.

---

psoriasis:

a **chronic**, occasionally **acute**, non-contagious - relapsing skin Dis-ease - distinct - reddish - slightly raised plaques or small round skin elevations covered with scales itching is seldom severe, and the lesions heal without scarring - **psoriasis** usually involves the **scalp - elbows - knees - back - buttocks** - occasionally generalised - p**soriasis** is an abnormally high rate of **mitosis** in the epidermal cells that maybe related to a substance carried in the blood - a defect in the **immune system** - or a **virus triggering factors** such as **trauma - infections - certain drugs** such as

(**beta-blockers - lithium**) **seasonal - hormonal** changes, **emotional stress** may initiate and intensify the condition; orthodox medical treatment is steroid ointment - natural sunlight - tar preparations - retinoids (chemicals similar to vitamin A) PUVA, a therapy that combines psoralen (chemical that increases the skins reaction to light); and artificial UV light; and a newly approved drug called (tegison); some evidence suggests that PUVA may increase the long-term risk of developing **2** usually nonfatal skin cancers (**squamous and basal cell**).

Use **anti-inflammatant-agents - antiallergenic-agents** to help alleviate conditions - effective **1%** solution **aloe vera.**

anti-inflammatant-essences:

use **anti-inflammatant-agents** to reduce the **pain** and **swelling** of inflammation.

[s]***ammi visnaga**	[s]***amyris**	[st]***angelica root**	[st]***artemesia** arborescens
[s]***bergamot**	[n]***calendula**	[st]***cedarwood atlas**	[s] celery seed
[s]***chamomiles**	[s] clary sage	[st]***eucalyptus** radiata	[s] guaiacwood
[s] helichrysum	[s] immortelle	[s] inula	[s]***lavender**
[st]***myrrh**	[s] patchouli	[st]***peppermint**	[st] pine needles
[s] rose	[s] sandalwood	[st] santolina	[s] tagetes
[st] turmeric	[st] yarrow.		
[st]***swt fennel seed;**	(prevents **toxic waste build-up** in body preceding inflammatory joint conditions)		
[st]***artemesia** arbores	(high content of azulene, highly effective eczema, **1%** solution > **aloe vera** gel).		

<u>antiallergenic-essences</u>:

use these **antiallergenic-agents** to reduce the effects of allergens.

[s] benzoin	[s] bergamot	[n] birch bud	[st] cajeputi
[st] carrot seed	[s] cedarwood atlas	[s]***chamomiles**	[n] geranium
[b] hyssop	[st] pine needles	[s] neroli	[st] tea tree.
<u>asthma:</u>	[st]***khellin**	(ammi visnaga).	
<u>general:</u>	[s] immortelle	[s] chamomile	[s] melissa	[st] yarrow.
<u>skin:</u>	[s] german chamomile	[s] melissa	[s] rose.
<u>sensitive skin:</u>	[st]***artemesia** arb;	(high azulene, effective eczema, **1**% solution > **aloe vera** gel)	
<u>dry eczema:</u>	[st] rose geranium	[s] sandalwood	[st] tea tree.
<u>weeping eczema:</u>	[st] juniper berry	[s] lavender	[st] myrrh.

---

scabies:

use **antipruritic-agents** for the relief of **scabies** and **itchmite bites**.

<u>antipruritic-essences</u>:

use **antipruritic-agents** to relieve **severe itching**.

[s] bergamot	[st]***black pepper**	[st] carrot seed	[s]***chamomile**
[s] clary sage	[s] inula	[s] lavender	[n]***lemon**
[s] patchouli	[st]***peppermint**	[st]***pine needles**	[st]***spearmint**
[st] tea tree	[rub] terebinth.		

<u>excellent cold blend</u>**:**	(peppermint - spearmint)		
[**st**] aniseed	[**st**]*****pine needles**	[**st**]*****spearmint**	[**st**]*****peppermint**.
[**st**] rosemary;	(kills lice and scabies).		
[**st**] aniseed;	(controls scabies and itch mite).		
[**st**] cinnamon;	(use direct to kill lice and scabies).		
[**st**] tea tree.			

<u>scarring</u>:

to reduce scarring of wounds - acne - use **vitamin** E - **vitamin** A - **wheatgerm** or **sesame seed** -**rosehip seed** oils.

use **cytophylactic-agents** - **cicatrisant-agents**.

<u>cicatrisant-agents</u>:

helps with the **formation** of **healthy scar tissue**.

<u>cicatrisant-essences</u>:

[s] benzoin tincture	[s] bergamot	[**st**] cajeputi	[s] chamomiles
[**st**] clove bud	[s] cypress	[**st**] eucalyptus radiata	[s] frankencense
[**st**] garlic	[**n**] geranium	[s] hypericum	[**b**] hyssop
[s] jasmine	[**st**] juniper berry	[**st**] lavandin	[s]*****lavender**
[**n**] lemon	[s] swt marjoram	[s] myrrh	[**st**] niaouli
[s] patchouli	[**st**] rose geranium	[**st**] rosemary	[**n**] common sage
[**st**] tea tree	[**rub**] terebinth	[**st**] swt thyme	[**st**] yarrow.

[**st**]*****artemesia** arborescens… (amazing results with **actinic keratosis**).

cytophylactic-agents:

these are **cellular regenerators** - helps in the **formation of new tissue cells**.

cytophylactic-essences:

helps in the regeneration of new tissue cells,

[st]***artemesia**	[st]***carrot seed**	[s] clary sage	[s]***frankencense**
[n] geranium	[s]***helichrysum**	[s] immortelle	[s]***lavender**
[s] mandarin	[s]***neroli**	[st]***palmarosa**	[s] patchouli
[s]***rose**	[st] rose geranium	[eu] spikenard	[s] tagetes
[s]***tangerine**	[st]***tea tree**.		

best essence:

[s]***swt orange**.

carrier oils:

vitamin A – **vitamin** E – **meadowfoam** – **rosehip seed** – **sesame seed** – **wheatgerm** oils.

---

scleroderma: or (**acrosclerosis**) scleroderma and wounds which do not heal.

scleroderma, also known as **systemic sclerosis**, is a chronic autoimmune disease characterised by the hardening (**sclero**) of the skin (**derma**). A hardening with loss of elasticity of the tissues – the skin maybe thickened, hardened, or pigmented patches ~ generalised or limited to extremities and or face (**acrosclerosis**).

limited scleroderma involves s manifestations that mainly affect the hands, arms and face.

In the more severe form, it also affects internal organs ie; kidneys, oesophagus, (leading to difficulty in swallowing) heart and or lungs. Prognosis is generally good for **limited cutaneous scleroderma** persons who escape lung complications, but is worse for those with the **diffuse cutaneous disease**, particularly in older age and for males.

Death occurs most often from lung, heart or kidney complications.

It is an **autoimmune Dis-ease condition**, in which the body's immune system attacks healthy tissues.

There are pure essential plant essences which may be beneficial in helping retain the **skins elasticity**.

antisclerotic-essences:

prevents the hardening of the tissue due to chronic inflammation.

[st] garlic   [n]*lemon.

elasticity-essences:

[st] swt basil	[s] benzoin	[st] carrot seed	[s] chamomiles
[s] frankencense	[s]*jasmine	[s]*lavender	[st] lemongrass
[s] linden blossom	[s]*mandarin	[st] myrrh	[s] neroli
[s] rose	[eu] spikenard.		

best combination:

[s]*jasmine   [s]*mandarin   [s]*lavender.

returns skin colour:

[s]*tangerine.

dry-mature-ageing:

[eu] spikenard   [s] vetivert.

puffiness:

[s] celery seed   [st] swt fennel seed.

wrinkles:

[st] carrot seed	[s] clary sage	[st] swt fennel seed	[s] frankencense
[n] geranium	[s] guaiacwood	[s] helichrysum	[s] jasmine
[n] lemon	[s] palmarosa	[s] patchouli	[s] rose
[st] rose geranium	[st] rosewood	[s] sandalwood	[eu] spikenard
[s] tangerine	[s] vetivert	[s] ylang-ylang.	

carrier oils:

vitamin A * vitamin E * rosehip * sesame * wheatgerm * jojoba * and / or meadowfoam oils.

---

seborrhoea:

a buildup of **sebum** within the hair follicles - preventing healthy skin and hair growth.

sebum-balancer-essences:

[s] lavender   [s] neroli   [st] palmarosa.

congested skin:

| [st] swt basil | [s] bergamot | [n] birch bud | [st] carrot seed |
| [s] cedarwood atlas | [s] clary sage | [s] elemi | [n] geranium |

[n] hypericum	[n]*jojoba	[st] juniper berry	[s] lavender (**tonic**)
[n] lemon	[st] lemongrass	[st] nutmeg	[st] palmarosa
[st] rosemary	[st] swt thyme	[st]*yarrow	[s]*ylang-ylang.

carrier oils:

jojoba * **meadowfoam** * **macadamia** oils.

---

sebum:

sebum is a mixture of **fats - cholesterol - proteins - inorganic salts** - sebum helps keep hair from drying - becoming brittle - forms a protective film to prevent excessive evaporation of water from the skin - keeps skin soft - pliable - inhibits the growth of certain bacteria - a secretion of sebaceous gland.

sebum-balancer-essences:

[st]*swt basil	[n]*geranium	[s]*ylang-ylang.
[s] lavender	[s] neroli	[st] palmarosa.

carrier oils:

jojoba * **meadowfoam** * **macadamia** oils.   (An excellent blend for correcting an imbalance).

---

shingles:

pain associated with peripheral nerve pain - dormant **herpes virus**, a legacy of chicken pox ~ viruses are invading agents responsible for most **epidemic illnesses**, includes influenza - colds - chicken pox - small pox - poliomyelitis - measles - also a many great vague undiagnosed fevers - many instances of diarrhoea are due to viral infections ~ some forms of pneumonia originate from viral - while others are **bacterial**.

antiviral-essences:

use **antiviral-agents** which kill viral organisms.

[**st**] artemesia / annua	[s]***bergamot**	[s] elemi	[**st**]***garlic**
[**st**] eucalyptus radiata	[**n**] geranium	[s] helichrysum	[s] immortelle
[s] lavender	[**st**] spike lavender	[**n**] lemon	[**n**] lime
[s] melissa	[**st**] origanum	[**st**] palmarosa	[s] rose, bulgarian
[**st**]***tea tree**	[**st**] sweet thyme.		

best antiviral-essences:

[s]***bergamot**;	(is a very powerful **antiviral** essence).
[**st**]***tea tree**;	(very powerful, well-known immune response stimulant to infection).
[**st**] eucalyptus;	(is not as powerful as **tea tree**)
<u>mediums</u>:	**baths - vapourisation - inhalants -** these are the best forms of applications).
<u>bath</u>:	(add a few antiviral essences to running bath water prior to emerging).
<u>steam inhalant</u>:	(steam inhalants best medium, due to fever accompanying a cold influenza etc).
<u>vapouriser</u>:	(whether a burner - electrical fragrancer - aerosol diffuser - not only helps **client**, but the best ways of reducing airborne transmission of infection to other members of the family).
<u>massage</u>:	**massage is contra-indicated to a fever**

antipruritic-essences:

[**st**] swt basil	[s] chamomiles	[s] lavender	[**n**]***lemon**
[s] inula	[**st**]***peppermint**	[**st**] pine needles	[**st**]***spearmint**
[**st**] tea tree	[**rub**] terebinth.		

snake bites:

antivenomous essences neutralises snake venom.

antivenomous-essences:

use **antivenomous-essences** - antivenoms neutralises poisons.

[st]***angelica root**;	(apply neat - helps in removing toxins from circulatory system).
[st]***swt fennel seed**	
[s] patchouli.	

snake bites:

[st]***angelica root**;	use neat to wound.

detoxify-circulatory system:

[st]***swt basil**	[st] sweet thyme.
[st]***swt fennel seed**;	(helps in removing toxins from circulatory system).

---

stretchmarks:

use **cicatrisant-agents - elasticity-agents**.

cicatrisant-essences:

[s] benzoin tincture	[s] bergamot	[st] cajeputi	[s] chamomiles
[st] clove bud	[s] cypress	[st] eucalyptus radiata	[s] frankencense

[st] garlic	[n] geranium	[s] hypericum	[b] hyssop
[s] jasmine	[st] juniper berry	[st] lavandin	[s]***lavender**
[n] lemon	[s] mandarin	[s] swt marjoram	[s] myrrh
[s] neroli	[st] niaouli	[s] patchouli	[s] rose
[st] rose geranium	[st] rosemary	[n] common sage	[s] tangerine
[st] tea tree	[rub] terebinth	[st] swt thyme	[st] yarrow.

[st]***artemesia** arbores; (amazing results with actinic keratosis).

elasticity-essences:

[st] swt basil	[s] benzoin	[st] carrot seed	[s] chamomiles
[s] frankencense	[s]***jasmine**	[s]***lavender**	[st] lemongrass
[s] linden blossom	[s]***mandarin**	[st] myrrh	[s] neroli
[s] rose.			

best combination: [s]***jasmine** [s]***mandarin** [s]***lavender**.

returns skin colour: [s]***tangerine**.

dry-mature-aging skin: [s] vetivert.

puffiness: [s] celery seed [st] swt fennel seed.

wrinkles:

[st] carrot seed	[s] clary sage	[st] swt fennel seed	[s] frankencense
[n] geranium	[s] guaiacwood	[s] helichrysum	[s] jasmine
[n] lemon	[st] palmarosa	[s] patchouli	[s] rose
[st] rose geranium	[st] rosewood	[s] sandalwood	[eu] spikenard
[s] tangerine	[s] vetivert	[s] ylang-ylang.	

carrier-oils:

vitamin A - **vitamin** E - **rosehip** - **sesame seed** - **jojoba** - **wheatgerm** oils. ~ preferred **jojoba** oil – **meadowfoam** oil.

---

sunburn:

is an injury to the skin due to acute, prolonged exposure to sun's UV rays, the damage to the skin cells caused by sun burn is due to inhibition of DNA and RNA synthesis, this leads to skin cell death - there may also be blood vessel damage as well as other structures in the dermis. Over-exposure to sunlight for years may result in leathery **skin texture - wrinkles - skin-folds - sagging skin - warty growth called keratosis - freckling** - yellow discolouration due to **abnormal elastic tissue, premature ageing** of the skin, as well as skin cancer.

suggested-essences to use are:

analgesics – anti-inflammatants – cicatrisant – cytophylactics – rejuvenators.

[st]*artemesia arborescens - > 1% aloe vera gel		(for sunburn and severely damaged cellular tissue).	
[n]*aloe vera gel	[s] roman chamomile	[st] eucalyptus radiata	[s]*lavender
[n] jojoba	[n] lemon	[st] niaouli.	

analgesic-essences:

are used for speedy pain relieving ie; **headaches - migraine - toothache - muscular aches - pains.**

add to bath - local massage blend or a compress on affected area.

[st] aniseed;	**1-2** drops on a compress for headache or stomach-ache.		
[st]*swt basil	[st] bay laurel	[s] benzoin	[s]*bergamot
[n] birch bud	[st]*black pepper	[st] cajeputi	[st] camphor

[s]***chamomiles**	[st] clove bud	[st] coriander	[s] elemi
[st] eucalyptus radiata	[st] galbanum	[st] garlic	[n] geranium
[st]***ginger**	[s] helichrysum	[st] lavandin	[s]***lavender**
[st] spike lavender	[s]***swt marjoram**	[st] niaouli	[st] nutmeg
[st] origanum	[st]***peppermint**	[st] pimento	[st] rose geranium
[st] rosemary	[st] rosewood	[rub] terebinth	[s] violet leaf
[st] yarrow.			

<u>anti-inflammatant-essences</u>:

reduces the **pain - swelling** of inflammation.

[s]***ammi visnaga**	[s]***amyris**	[st]***angelica root**	[st]***artemesia** arborescens
[s]***bergamot**	[n]***calendula**	[st]***cedarwood atlas**	[s] celery seed
[s]***chamomiles**	[s] clary sage	[st]***eucalyptus radiata**	[s] guaiacwood
[s] helichrysum	[s] immortelle	[s] inula	[s]***lavender**
[st]***myrrh**	[s] patchouli	[st]***peppermint**	[st] pine needles
[s] rose	[s] sandalwood	[st] santolina	[s] tagetes
[st] turmeric	[st] yarrow.		
[st]***swt fennel seed**;	(prevents **toxic waste build-up** which precedes inflammatory joint conditions).		

<u>cicatrisant-essences</u>:

[s] benzoin tincture	[s] bergamot	[st] cajeputi	[s] chamomiles
[st] clove bud	[s] cypress	[st] eucalyptus radiata	[s] frankencense

[**st**] garlic	[**n**] geranium	[s] hypericum	[**b**] hyssop
[s] jasmine	[**st**] juniper berry	[**st**] lavandin	[s]***lavender**
[**n**] lemon	[**n**] mandarin	[s] sweet marjoram	[s] myrrh
[s] neroli	[**st**] niaouli	[s] patchouli	[s] rose
[**st**] rose geranium	[**st**] rosemary	[**n**] common sage	[s] tangerine
[**st**] tea tree	[**rub**] terebinth	[**st**] sweet thyme	[**st**] yarrow.
[**st**]***artemesia arbores**;	(amazing results with **actinic keratosis**).		

<u>cytophylactic-essences</u>:

helps in the formation of new tissue cells.

[**st**]***artemesia** arbores	[**st**]***carrot seed**	[s] clary sage	[s]***frankencense**
[**n**] geranium	[**n**]***helichrysum**	[s] immortelle	[s]***lavender**
[s] mandarin	[s]***neroli**	[s]***sweet orange**	[**st**]***palmarosa**
[s] patchouli	[s]***rose**	[**st**] rose geranium	[**eu**] spikenard
[s] tagetes	[s]***tangerine**	[**st**]***tea tree**.	

<u>rejuvenator-essences</u>:

rejuvenator essences help in the **rejuvenation** of the **skin tissue**.

[s] benzoin	[**st**]***carrot seed**	[s] frankencense	[s] jasmine
[s] lavender	[**n**] lemon	[**st**] myrrh	[s] neroli
[s] patchouli	[**st**] peppermint	[**b**] pettitgrain	[s] rose
[**st**] rosemary	[s] sandalwood.		

sun tanning:

for use in sun tan preparations.

suggested-essences:

[n]*aloe vera   [n]*jojoba   [n]*lemon   [s]*bergamot
                                            (bergapten free)

[s]*swt orange   [st]*niaouli.

---

surface veins:

are broken surface capillaries which may result in - **leg ulcers** - **varicose veins** - **hereditary varicose veins** - **pregnancy varicose veins** - **chilblains** - **bad circulation** due to lack of exercise or stress related. Surface - thread or broken capillaries - are sometimes a problem for older women - **chamomile** and **rose essences** can help to diminish this problem - though it may take several months before a real improvement is seen.

use **astringents - vasoconstrictors - venous tonics - fat burner-agents:**

[st] carrot seed	[s]*roman chamomile	[s] mandarin	[s] neroli
[st] niaouli	[s] parsley herb	[s] rose.	
[s] rose;	(strengthens capillary walls).		
[n]*lemon;	(smooths out broken capillaries).		
[s]*neroli;	(a **skin rejuvenator** for thread veins ~ stretch marks).		
[s] cypress;	(cause capillaries to contract locally - helpful in cases of heat - inflammation - redness).		

astringent-essences:

contracts, tightens - binds the tissues - reduces and / or balances excessive fluid loss.

astringent without drying = **balances** oily skin - contracts - tightens - softens phlegm.

[st] bay laurel	[s] benzoin	[n] birch bud	[s]***cedar-wood** atlas
[st] caraway seed	[s]***cypress**	[s]***franken-cense**	[n] geranium
[s] guaiacwood	[s] helichrysum	[s] hypericum	[b] hyssop
[s] immortelle	[st]***juniper berry**	[n]***lemon**	[n] lime
[s] linden blossom	[st] litsea cubeba	[st]***myrrh**	[n] myrtle
[s] oakmoss	[s] patchouli	[st] peppermint	[s] rose
[st] rose geranium	[st] rosemary	[n] common sage	[s]***sandal-wood** [st] yarrow.

<u>circulation</u>: (excellent for all types of excess bleeding - haemorrhage).

<u>reproductive</u>: (inhibits uterine haemorrhage).

<u>inflammation</u>: (breasts = excessive milk).

<u>congestion</u>: (of breasts whilst breast feeding).

<u>respiratory</u>: (makes mucus more fluid - easier to express, liquefies, removes from lungs).

<u>skin</u>: (balancing to oily skin).

vasoconstrictor-essences:

contracts, tightens and binds the tissues - reduces and / or balances excessive fluid loss - **astringent** without drying = **balances** oily skin, contracts - tightens blood vessel walls.

[s] cypress	[n] geranium	[n] lemon	[st] peppermint
[st] rose geranium.			

venous tonic-essences:

are a **tonic** to the veins.

[n]*lemon.

fat burner-agents:

pure essential plant essences which helps in the reduction of bodily fats.

[st] swt basil	[s] bergamot	[st] black pepper	[st]*cardamom
[s] cypress	[st] swt fennel seed	[st] grapefruit	[st] juniper berry
[s]*lavender	[n]*lemon	[st] lemongrass	[n] lime
[s] swt orange	[st] onion	[st] origanum	[b] pettitgrain
[st]*rosemary	[n] common sage	[st] swt thyme.	

treatment:

use in **massage blends - crèmes - lotions** apply daily - must be done regularly for best effect.

Treatment to continue for some time - best to alternate essences rather than use them all at the same time.

compress leg treatment:

<u>1</u> hour leg compress treatment.

use for **aching legs - puffy feet - ankles - leg problems - varicose veins**.

carrier oils:

5 ml each of **rosehip – vitamin** A **– vitamin** E **– avocado – jojoba – sunflower** or **wheatgerm** oils.

application:

1) **2** large pieces of gauze soaked in appropriate essential essences in cool water, (squeeze out)
2) bandage - wide crepe bandages, long enough to cover leg from ankle to above knee - lay **Client** on their back - with legs elevated enough to bandage - warn **Client** compresses maybe cold.
3) support the leg with one hand - wrap gauze diagonally with the other hand - keep leg supported - starting with foot - wrap bandage around to cover compresses.
4) make sure leg is supported - especially under the knee.
5) leave each leg for **15** minutes same for varicosed legs.
6) support leg and unwrap - treat the other leg in the same way.
7) dry - finish treatment here or continue with leg and back massage.

leg cramps:

massage legs with upwards strokes before retiring for the night.

[**n**] lemon;	(hypertension)	8 drops
[**st**] rosemary;	(hypotension)	10 drops
[s] lavender;		5 drops
[**n**] common sage;		3 drops
[s] swt marjoram;		10 drops.

<u>application</u>:	(5 mls each of **evening primrose - hazelnut - calendula - hypericum - rosehip - carrot root - sesame - sunflower - vitamin** A - E **- wheatgerm** oils). (Then apply **IP essence** enriched crème).
<u>suitable carrier oils</u>:	**rosehip - vitamin** E - A **- avocado - jojoba - sunflower - wheatgerm** oils.

---

systemic lupus erythematosus:

SLE, or **lupus**, is an **auto-immune, inflammatory** dis-ease of the connective tissue, occurs mostly in young women of reproductive years. Autoimmune dis-ease is where the body attacks its own tissues ~ failing to differentiate between what is foreign and what is not. In SLE, damage to blood vessel walls results in the release of chemicals which mediate the inflammatory response. Blood vessel damage maybe associated with virtually everybody system. Cause is unknown as yet, its onset being gradual to abrupt. Not contagious, but thought to be hereditary. There is evidence of other connective disorders --- especially **rheumatoid arthritis, rheumatic fever**, in relatives of SLE victims. The Dis-ease maybe triggered by medications, such as **penicillin, sulpha**, or **tetracycline**, exposure to **excessive sunlight, injury, emotional** upset, **infections**, or other **stress** ~ once these are recognised, these triggering factors must be avoided.

<u>symptoms</u>: recognition of **systemic lupus**, is obvious when patient (**particularly young woman**) has a febrile Dis-ease with an erythematous skin rash, polyarthritis, evidence of renal dis-ease, intermittent pleuritic pain, leukopenia, and hyperglobulinemia with anti-DNA antibodies. SLE can be difficult to differentiate from other connective tissue disorders in its early stages; eg; maybe mistaken for **rheumatoid arthritis**, if arthritic symptoms predominate.

Meticulous evaluation and long-term observation maybe required before the diagnosis is established - **migraine, epilepsy**, or **psychoses** maybe initial findings - patients with **discoid lesions** must be evaluated to differentiate **discoid** from **systemic lupus**, - **painful joints - low grade fevers - fatigue - mouth ulcers - weight loss - enlarged lymph nodes - spleen - photosensitivity - rapid loss** of large amounts of scalp hair and sometimes eruptions, called '**butterfly rash**' across the bridge of the nose - other skin lesions may occur with blistering and ulcerations.

The terminology `lupus`, derives from the likeness of the **systemic lupus erythematous** skin lesions to that of resembling the damage by the bite of a wolf - the most serious complications of 'lupus' are inflammation of the **heart - liver - spleen - kidneys - lungs** also the **central nervous system** - some **drugs** including;

(hydralazine - procainamide - beta blockers) produce positive ANA tests - occasionally, **lupus-like** syndrome. These features disappear if the drug is withdrawn promptly.

The American Rheumatism Association has proposed criteria for classification, (but not diagnosis) of SLE;

<u>four of the following are required</u>:

1) malar rash;
2) discoid rash;
3) photosensitivity;
4) oral ulceration;
5) arthritis;
6) serositis;
7) renal disorder; (< 1500/uL), **haemolytic anaemia**;
8) leukopenia; (< 4000/uL) **lymphopenia thrombocytopenia** (< 100,000uL)
9) neurological disorder; antibody or a false-positive STS;
10) positive LE cell or anti-DNA or anti-Sm.
11) antinuclear antibodies in raised titer.

Mixed connective tissue Dis-ease, MCTD, is a syndrome with clinical features of systemic lupus erythematous overlapping with those of progressive **systemic sclerosis** and **polio myositis / dermatomyositis**.

<u>suggested-essences</u>:

tinea:

for the relief of tinea - kills and or inhibits the growth of yeasts - moulds - candida etc.

use **antifungal-essences** in a topical application.

antifungal-essences:

[st] angelica root	[n]***calendula**	[st] camphor	[s] cedarwood atlas
[st] coriander	[st] cinnamon leaf	[st] citronella	[s] elemi
[st] swt fennel seed	[st] garlic	[s]***helichrysum**	[s] hypericum
[s] immortelle	[s] lavender	[st] lemongrass	[s] swt marjoram
[st]***myrrh**	[st] nutmeg	[s] patchouli	[n] common sage
[st] savory	[s] tagetes	[st]***tea tree**	[st]***swt thyme**.

---

urticaria:

a skin reaction to **certain foods - drugs** - or any **substance** which may produce a **severe allergic reaction** - creating inflammation and hives - use **antiallergenic-agents - anti-inflammatant-agents - antipruritic-agents.**

antiallergenic-essences:

use these **antiallergenic-essences** to reduce the effects of **allergens**.

[s] benzoin	[s] bergamot	[n] birch bud	[st] artemesia arborescens
[st] cajeputi	[st] carrot seed	[s] cedarwood atlas	[s]***roman chamomile**
[s] german chamomile	[n] geranium	[b] hyssop	[s] immortelle

[st] juniper berry	[st]**khellin	[s] lavender	[s]*melissa
[st] myrrh	[s] neroli	[st] pine needles	[s]*rose
[st] rose geranium	[s] sandalwood	[st] tea tree	[st] yarrow.

asthma: [st]**khellin.

general: [s] immortelle [s] chamomile [s] melissa [st] yarrow.

skin: [s] german chamomile [st] artemesia arbores. [s]*melissa [s]*rose.

asthma: [s]*ammi visnaga.

sensitive skin: [st] artemesia arborescens.

anti-inflammatant-essences:

reduces the **pain** and **swelling** of inflammation.

[s]*ammi visnaga	[s]*amyris	[st]*angelica root	[st]*artemesia arborescens
[st] aniseed	[s]*bergamot	[n]*calendula	[st]*cedarwood atlas
[s] celery seed	[s]*chamomiles	[s] clary sage	[st]*eucalyptus radiata
[s] guaiacwood	[s] helichrysum	[s] immortelle	[s] inula
[s]*lavender	[st]*myrrh	[s] patchouli	[st]*peppermint
[st] pine needles	[s] rose	[s] sandalwood	[st] santolina
[s] tagetes	[st] turmeric	[st] yarrow.	

[st]*swt fennel seed; (prevents toxic waste build-up in body which precedes inflammatory conditions).

antipruritic-essences:

use **antipruritic-agents** to relieve **severe itching**.

[s] bergamot	[**st**]***black pepper**	[**st**] carrot seed	[s]***chamomile**
[s] clary sage	[s] inula	[s] lavender	[**n**]***lemon**
[s] patchouli	[**st**]***peppermint**	[**st**]***pine needles**	[**st**]***spearmint**
[**st**] tea tree	[**rub**] terebinth.		
[**st**] rosemary;	(kills lice and scabies).		
[**st**] aniseed;	(controls scabies and itch mite).		
[**st**] cinnamon;	(use direct to kill lice and scabies).		

warts:

which are masses produced by uncontrolled growths of epithelial skin cells; a virus (**papillomavirus**) most warts are non-cancerous ~ **escharotic-agents** are used for the treating and removal of warts.

escharotic-essences:

[**st**]***cinna-mon leaf**	[**st**] garlic	[s] lavender	[**n**] lemon	[**st**] santolina.

Aromatherapy treatment:

applications consist of topical application of **antiviral-essences** to the wart, a thin layer of vege gel or similar non-toxic gel for preventing the concentrated pure essential essences from coming into contact with the healthy skin - cover with a bandaid, re-apply periodically.

orthodox medical treatment:

may involve cryosurgery with **liquid nitrogen - electrosurgery - chemical destruction - injections - carbon dioxide - laser surgery - surgical excision - or immunotherapy.**

antiviral-essences:

use **antiviral-agents** for the removal of warts.

[st] carrot seed	***castor oil**	[s]*cinnamon leaf	[st] clove bud
[st]*garlic	[s] lavender	[n]*lemon	[st] onion
[st] santolina	[st] thuja. +	* castor oil.	

---

weight loss:

some pure essential plant essences which are valuable in the reduction of body fats.

fat-burner-essences:

[st] swt basil	[st] black pepper	[st] cardamom	[s] cypress
[st] **swt fennel seed**	[st] grapefruit	[st] juniper berry	[s] lavender
[s] swt orange	[st] lemongrass	[n] lime	[st] onion
[b] pettitgrain	[st] rosemary	[n] common sage	[st] swt thyme

medium: **massage - local body rub.**

(best used in a massage blend and vigorous local rub to affected areas of the body.

---

windburn:

sunburn damage from the wind whilst in the sunshine, can be quite severe.

suggested-essences:

[s] roman chamomile	[s] lavender

wounds:

for clean, healthy wound healing - use **cicatrisant-agents** - **cytophylactic-agents**.

cicatrisant-essences:

cicatrisant essences helps in the formation of **scar tissue**.

[s] bergamot	[st] cajeputi	[s] chamomiles	[st] clove bud
[s] cypress	[st] eucalyptus radiata	[s] frankencense	[st] garlic
[n] geranium	[s] hypericum	[b] hyssop	[s] jasmine
[st] juniper berry	[st] lavandin	[s] lavender	[n] lemon
[st] niaouli	[s] patchouli	[st] rose geranium	[st] rosemary
[n] common sage	[st] tea tree	[rub] terebinth	[st] swt thyme
[st] yarrow.			

[st]***artemesia arbores**;   (produces some amazing results - **actinic keratosis**).

cytophylactic-essences:

cellular regenerators - vital for growth and in the formation of new tissue cells.

[st]***artemesia**	[st]***carrot seed**	[s] clary sage	[s]***frankencense**
[n] geranium	[s]***helichrysum**	[s]***lavender**	[s] mandarin
[s]***neroli**	[s]****swt orange**	[st]***palmarosa**	[s] patchouli
[s]***rose**	[st]***rose geranium**	[eu] spikenard	[s] tagetes
[s]***tangerine**	[st]***tea tree**.		

carrier oils: **vitamin**-A * **vitamin**-E * **rosehip seed** * **sesame seed** * **meadowfoam** oils.

x-ray protection:

protection from x-ray frequencies -- apply local application to the skin prior to treatment - will lessen the effects of the rays.

[s]**lavender** [s]**neroli**.

THERAPEUTIC ACTIONS for the   (part two)   56
INTEGUMENTARY IMBALANCES:

antiageing	antiallergenics	antibiotics	antifungal	anti-inflammatant
antipruritic	antisclerotics	antiscorbutic	antiseptic	antisudorific
antivenomous	antiviral	arterial vaso-dilator	astringents	bactericidal
bacteriostatic	cicatrisant	cobalt therapy	collagen treatment	cytophylactic
deodourant	disinfectant	emollient	eye-muscle-strengthener escharotics	
facial-capillary-treat	haemostatic	hair-growth-stimulant	hair tonic	hydrating-essence
hypersensitivity	insecticide	insect repellents	parasiticide	penetrating-oil
photo-toxic	preservative	prophylactic	radiation-antidote	rejuvenator-skin
rehydration	resolvent	rubefacient	skin cleanser	skin-glands
skin-photo-sensitisation	skin-tone	skin-types	styptic	sudorific
tissue stimulant	vasoconstrictor	vasodilator	venous-tonic	vulnerary
weight loss.				

antiageing-agents:

are agents which rejuvenate the tissues.

rejuvenator-essences:

[s] clary sage	[s] cypress	[s] frankincense	[s] guaiacwood
[**n**] geranium	[s] helichrysum	[s] jasmine	[**n**]***lemon**
[s] linden blossom	[**eu**]***spikenard**	[**st**] sweet thyme.	

for ageing skin – congestive skin – elasticity – wrinkles:

| [**n**]***lemon** | [**st**] onion | [**eu**]***spikenard** | [**st**] swt thyme. |

---

antiallergenic-agents:

antiallergenics reduce the effects of **allergens** use to reduce effects of **allergens**.

antiallergenic-essences:

use these **antiallergenic-essences** to reduce the effects of **allergens**.

[s] benzoin	[s] bergamot	[**n**] birch bud	[**st**] artemesia arborescens
[**st**] cajeputi	[**st**] carrot seed	[s] cedarwood atlas	[s]***roman chamomile**
[s] german chamomile	[**n**] geranium	[**b**] hyssop	[s] immortelle
[**st**] juniper berry	[**st**]****khellin**	[s] lavender	[s]***melissa**
[**st**] myrrh	[s] neroli	[**st**] pine needles	[s]***rose**
[**st**] rose geranium	[s] sandalwood	[**st**] tea tree	[**st**] yarrow.

asthma:

[**st**]****khellin**.

general:	[s] immortelle	[s] chamomile	[s] melissa [st] yarrow.
skin:	[s] german chamomile	[st] artemesia arbores.	[s]*melissa [s]*rose.
dry eczema:	[st] rose geranium	[s] sandalwood	[st] tea tree.
weeping eczema:	[st] juniper berry	[s] lavender	[st] myrrh.
sensitive skin:	[st]*artemesia;	(contains high azulene, highly effective eczema 1% > aloe vera gel).	
mediums:	**bath - steam inhalation - massage - local rub - inhale - vapouriser - diffusor.**		
bath:	(add a few drops to running bath water, prior to emerging, make sure mixed well).		
steam inhalation:	(add a few drops to bowl hot water - cover head with towel - inhale few minutes).		
massage:	(add a few drops to full-body massage blend).		
local rub:	(maybe applied to a chest rub - a hand - or back rub)		
inhale:	(maybe inhaled off a tissue or handkerchief)		
vapouriser:	(add a few drops to water to burn in a vapouriser)		
diffusor:	(or a diffusor, whichever is most suitable medium for your **clients** benefit).		

---

antibiotic-agents:

fights infections in the body.

[s] angelica root	[st] garlic	[s] lavender	[st] niaouli
[st] myrrh	[st] tea tree.		

antifungal-agents:

essential essences are used to kill and / or inhibit the growth of **yeasts - moulds - candida** etc.

<u>antifungal-essences</u>:

[**st**] angelica root	[**n**]***calendula**	[**st**] camphor	[s] cedarwood atlas
[**st**] coriander	[**st**] cinnamon leaf	[**st**] citronella	[s] elemi
[**st**] swt fennel seed	[**st**] garlic	[s]***helichrysum**	[**n**] hypericum
[s] immortelle	[s] lavender	[**st**] lemongrass	[s] swt marjoram.
[**st**]***myrrh**	[**st**] nutmeg	[s] patchouli	[**st**] savory
[s] tagetes	[**st**]***tea tree**	[st]***swt thyme**.	

---

anti-inflammatant-agents:

reduces the pain and swelling of inflammation.

<u>anti-inflammatant-essences</u>:

[s]***amyris**	[**st**]***angelica root**	[**st**]***artemesia** arbores	[s]***bergamot**
[**n**]***calendula**	[s] celery seed	[s]***chamomiles**	[s] clary sage
[**st**]***eucalyptus** radiata	[s] guaiacwood	[s] helichrysum	[s] immortelle
[s] inula	[s]***khellin**	[s]***lavender**	[s] melissa
[**st**]***myrrh**	[s] patchouli	[**st**]***peppermint**	[**st**] pine needles
[s] rose	[s] sandalwood	[**st**] santolina	[s] tagetes
[**st**] turmeric	[**st**] yarrow.		
[**st**]***swt fennel seed;**	(prevents **toxic waste build-up** in body preceding inflammatory joint conditions).		

antipruritic-agents:

using **antipruritic** essences to relieve the severe itching.

antipruritic-essences:

[s]***bergamot**	[st]***black pepper**	[s]***chamomiles**	[s] inula
[s] lavender	[n]***lemon**	[st]***peppermint**	[st]***pine needles**
[st]***spearmint**	[st]***tea tree**	[rub] terebinth.	
[st]***peppermint** +	[st]***spearmint**;	(makes an excellent cold blend)	

---

antisclerotic-agents:

prevents the hardening of the tissue due to chronic inflammation.

antisclerotic-essences:

[**st**] garlic   [n]***lemon**.

---

antiscorbutic-agents:

prevents scurvy - the deficiency of **vitamin** C.

antiscorbutic-essences:

[s] fir needles   [**st**] ginger   [n]***lemon**   [n]***lime**.

---

antiseptic-agents:

helps in **preventing tissue degeneration** - all pure essential plant essences **inhibit** the growth of organisms - **bacteria** - **germs**, some essential essences being more effective than others, best indicated by*.

antiseptic-essences:

- [s] amyris
- [n] birch bud
- [s] cedarwood atlas
- [s] clary sage
- [st]*eucalyptus radiata
- [n] geranium
- [b] hyssop
- [s]*lavender
- [n] lime
- [n] myrtle
- [st] origanum
- [st] peppermint
- [st]*rosemary
- [s] tagetes
- [st] swt thyme
- [st] yarrow
- [st] bay laurel
- [st] black pepper
- [s] german chamomile
- [st] clove bud
- [st] sweet fennel seed
- [st] ginger
- [s] jasmine
- [st] spike lavender
- [s] sweet marjoram
- [st] niaouli
- [st] palmarosa
- [st] pine needles
- [st] rosewood
- [s] tangerine
- [s] verbena lemon
- [s] ylang-ylang.
- [s] benzoin
- [st] cajeputi
- [s] roman chamomile
- [st] cumin
- [s] fir needles
- [st] grapefruit
- [st]*juniper berry
- [n] lemon
- [st] may chang
- [st] nutmeg
- [s] parsley herb
- [s] rose
- [s]*sandalwood
- [st] tarragon
- [s] vetivert
- [s]*bergamot
- [st] caraway seed
- [st] cinnamon leaf
- [s] cypress
- [s]*frankencense
- [s] helichrysum
- [st] lavandin
- [st] lemongrass
- [st] myrrh (thyroid)
- [s] swt orange
- [s] patchouli
- [st] rose geranium
- [eu] spikenard
- [st]*tea tree
- [s] violet leaf

<u>excretory antiseptic:</u> [st]*juniper berry.

---

antisudorific-agents:

pure essential essences which help in reducing sweating.

<u>antisudorific-essences:</u>

- [s] clary sage
- [s] cypress
- [s] elemi
- [n] common sage.

antivenomous-agents:

antivenom-agents neutralises poisons.

snake bites:	[st]*angelica root;	(use neat to wound).

detoxify-circ-system:

[st]*swt basil	[st] swt thyme.
[st]*swt fennel seed;	(helps in removing toxins from circulatory system).

---

antiviral-agents:

viruses are the invading agents responsible for most epidemic illnesses - including influenza - chicken pox - small pox - poliomyelitis - measles - colds - also a great many vague undiagnosed fevers - many instances of diarrhoea due to viral infections - some forms of pneumonia originate from viral - while others are bacterial.

use **antiviral agents** which kill viral organisms.

[st] artemesia annua	[s]*bergamot	[s] elemi	[st]*garlic
[n] geranium	[s] helichrysum	[s] immortelle	[st]*eucalyptus radiata
[s] lavender	[st] sweet lavender	[n] lemon	[n] lime
[s] melissa	[st] origanum	[st] palmarosa	[s] rose bulgarian
[st]*tea tree	[st] sweet thyme.		

<u>best antiviral-essences</u>:

[s]***bergamot**;	(is a very powerful **antiviral essence**).
[**st**]***tea tree**;	(very powerful, well known stimulant for immune response to infection).
[**st**] eucalyptus radiata;	(is **not as** powerful as **tea tree**.)
<u>mediums</u>:	**bath - vapour - inhalants** - these are the best forms of treatments for viruses).
<u>bath</u>:	(add a few drops to running bath water, prior to emerging, make sure mixed well).
<u>steam inhalant</u>:	(best medium, due to fever usually accompanying a cold, influenza etc)
<u>massage</u>:	(massage is **contra-indicated** with fever)
<u>inhale</u>:	(maybe inhaled off a tissue or handkerchief)
<u>vapouriser</u>:	(whether burner - electrical fragrancer - diffusor - or simply means of a few drops of pure essence on the light-globe - only helps **Client**, but one of the best ways of reducing air-borne transmission of infection to their family).

---

arterial-vasodilator-agents:

helps in opening up the arterial veins.

<u>vasodilator-essences</u>:

[**st**]***black pepper**   [**st**] garlic   [s] swt marjoram.

---

astringic-agents:

contracts, tightens and binds the tissues - reduces and / or balances excessive fluid loss – these essences are **astringent** without drying - balances oily skin – also contracts, tightens and softens phlegm.

astringic-essences:

contracts - tightens - binds the tissues.

[**st**] bay laurel	[s] benzoin	[**n**] birch bud	[s]***cedarwood atlas**
[**st**] caraway seed	[s] celery seed	[**st**] coriander	[s]***cypress**
[s] elemi	[s]***frankencense**	[**n**] geranium	[**st**] grapefruit
[s] guaiacwood	[s] helichrysum	[s] hypericum	[**b**] hyssop
[s] immortelle	[**st**]***juniper** berry	[**n**]***lemon**	[**n**] lime
[s] linden blossom	[s] litsea cubeba	[**st**]***khellin**	[**st**]***myrrh**
[**n**] myrtle	[s] patchouli	[**st**] peppermint	[s] rose
[**st**] rose geranium	[**st**] rosemary	[**n**] common sage	[s]***sandalwood**
[**st**] yarrow.			

circulation:	(excellent for all types of excess bleeding and haemorrhage).
reproductive:	(inhibits uterine haemorrhage).
inflammation:	(breasts - excessive milk).
congestion:	(of breasts whilst breast feeding).
respiratory:	(makes mucus more fluid and easier to express, liquefies, removes mucus from lungs).
skin:	(balancing to oily skin).

---

bactericidal-agents:

kills bacteria - most pure essential essences are **bactericidal** and **antiseptics**.

bactericidal-essences:

[**st**] swt basil	[s] benzoin	[s]***bergamot**	[s] chamomiles
[**st**]***cajeputi**	[**st**] cinnamon leaf	[**st**] cumin	[**st**]***clove bud**

[s] elemi	[st]*eucalyptus radiata	[st]*garlic	[s] helichrysum
[s] immortelle	[st]*juniper berry	[s]*lavender	[n]*lemon
[st] lemongrass	[n] lime	[st] litsea cubeba	[st]*myrrh (thyroid)
[n] myrtle	[s]*neroli	[st]*niaouli	[st] origanum
[st] palmarosa	[s] rose	[st]*rosemary	[st] rosewood
[s]*sandalwood	[st] spruce	[st]*tea tree	[st] swt thyme.

<u>spec/microbes:</u> (staphylococcus - streptococcus - gonococcus - pneumococcus)

<u>spec/microbe:</u> (staphylococcus aurens, ie; - **infected wounds - abscess - boils**).

<u>spec/essence:</u> [st]*tea tree.

<u>spec/microbes:</u> (streptococcus - gonococcus - pneumococcus).

<u>spec/essence:</u> [s]*sandalwood (- specific to - **kidney infections**)

<u>spec/essence:</u> [st]*swt thyme (- specific to - e. coli, some kidney infections).

<u>spec/essence:</u> [n] lemon (- specific to - **c. diphtheria**).

<u>spec/essence:</u> [st] cinnamon leaf (- specific to - **typhus bacillus**)

<u>spec/essence:</u> [st] clove bud (- specific to - **m. tuberculosis**)

*****Aromatherapists** will not deal with these dis-eases, but this list shows the plant essences effectiveness in **fighting** and **strengthening** the **immune system** against infectious dis-eases by attacking microbes.

<u>**bacteriostatic-agents:**</u>

all essential essences, particularly those listed under **antiseptics** and **bactericidals** inhibits bacteria growth.

antiseptic-essences:

helps in **preventing tissue degeneration** - all essential essences **inhibit** the growth of organisms bacteria and germs, some essential essences being more effective than others, best indicated by*.

[s] amyris	[st] swt basil	[st] bay laurel	[s] benzoin
[s]***bergamot**	[n] birch bud	[st] black pepper	[st] cajeputi
[st] camphor	[st] cardamom	[s] cedarwood atlas	[s] chamomiles
[st] cinnamon leaf	[s] clary sage	[st] clove bud	[n] common sage
[st] cumin	[s] cypress	[st]***eucalyptus** radiata	[st] swt fennel seed
[s] fir needles	[s]***frankencense**	[st] garlic	[n] geranium
[st] ginger	[st] grapefruit	[s] hypericum	[b] hyssop
[s] jasmine	[st]***juniper** berry	[st] lavandin	[s]***lavender**
[st] spike lavender	[n] lemon	[st] lemongrass	[n] lime
[st] litsea cubeba	[s] swt marjoram	[st] myrrh - (thyroid)	[n] myrtle
[s] neroli	[st] niaouli	[st] nutmeg	[s] swt orange
[st] origanum	[st] palmarosa	[s] parsley, herb	[s] patchouli
[st] peppermint	[st] pine needles	[s] rose	[st] rose geranium
[st]***rosemary**	[st] rosewood	[s]***sandalwood**	[s] tagetes
[s] tangerine	[st] tarragon	[st]***tea tree**	[rub] terebinth
[st] swt thyme	[s] verbena lemon	[s] vetivert	[s] violet leaf
[st] yarrow	[s] ylang-ylang.		

bactericidal-essences:

kills bacteria - most pure essential essences are **bactericidal** and **antiseptics**.

| [st] swt basil | [s] benzoin | [s]***bergamot** | [s] chamomiles |
| [st]***cajeputi** | [st] cinnamon leaf | [st] cumin | [st]***clove bud** |

[s] elemi	[**st**]***eucalyptus** radiata	[**st**]***garlic**	[s] helichrysum
[s] immortelle	[**st**]*juniper berry	[s]***lavender**	[**n**]***lemon**
[**st**] lemongrass	[**n**] lime	[**st**] litsea cubeba	[**st**]***myrrh** - (thyroid)
[**n**] myrtle	[s]***neroli**	[**st**]***niaouli**	[**st**] origanum
[**st**] palmarosa	[s] rose	[**st**]***rosemary**	[**st**] rosewood
[s]***sandalwood**	[**st**] spruce	[**st**]***tea tree**	[**st**] swt thyme.

---

cicatrisant-agents:

helps with the formation of healthy scar tissue.

cicatrisant-essences:

[s] benzoin tincture	[s] bergamot	[**st**] cajeputi	[s] chamomiles
[**st**] clove bud	[s] cypress	[**st**] eucalyptus radiata	[s] frankencense
[**st**] garlic	[**n**] geranium	[s] hypericum	[**b**] hyssop
[s] jasmine	[**st**] juniper berry	[**st**] lavandin	[s]***lavender**
[**n**]***lemon**	[s] swt marjoram	[s] myrrh	[**st**] niaouli
[s] patchouli	[**st**] rose geranium	[**st**] rosemary	[**n**] common sage
[**st**] tea tree	[**rub**] terebinth	[**st**] swt thyme	[**st**] yarrow.
[**st**]***artemesia** arbores;	(amazing results with **actinic keratosis**).		

---

cobalt therapy:

reducing the after-effects of radiation. (apply to skin prior to treatment)

[s]***lavender**   [s]***neroli**.

collagen formation:

swt orange essence has **cytophylactic** action for helping with the formation of collagen, vital for growth and repair of body tissue - has a sweating action, rids of toxins in congested skin, plumps out the tissue; hydrates, brings warmth, but also works for dry - wrinkled skin - dermatitis - an all-round skin tonic - apply locally for skin problems, use with **lemon juice** for tanning.

collagen-formation-essences:

[s]**swt orange.

mediums:	**steam inhalation - crèmes - lotions - face massage.**
steam inhalant:	add a few drops sweet orange essence to bowl very hot water - cover head with towel - inhale for a few minutes.
crèmes:	add to basic crème for use morning and evening.
lotions:	add a few drops to lotion for facial use.
facial massages:	have an Aromatherapy facial massage.

---

cytophylactic-agents:

these are cellular regenerators - helps in the formation of new tissue cells.

cytophylactic-essences:

helps in the regeneration of new tissue cells,

[st]***artemesia**	[st]*carrot seed	[s] clary sage	[s]***frankencense**
[n] geranium	[s]***helichrysum**	[s] immortelle	[s]***lavender**
[s] mandarin	[s]***neroli**	[st]***palmarosa**	[s] patchouli
[s]***rose**	[st] rose geranium	[eu] spikenard	[s] tagetes
[s]***tangerine**	[st]*tea tree.		

best essence:

[s]***swt orange**.

carrier oils:

vitamin A – vitamin E – meadowfoam – rosehip seed – sesame seed – wheatgerm oils.

mediums: **steam inhalant - crèmes - lotions - facial massages**.

---

deodourant-agents:

are used to destroy the bacteria causing the odour.

deodourant-essences:

destroys the **bacteria** causing the odour.

[s] benzoin	[s]***bergamot**	[st] citronella	[s]***clary sage**
[st] coriander	[s]***cypress**	[n] geranium	[st]***eucalyptus** radiata
[s]***lavender**	[st] lemongrass	[st] myrrh	[s]***neroli**
[s] patchouli	[b]***pettitgrain**	[st] pine needles	[st]***rose geranium**
[st]***rosewood**...			

---

disinfectant-agents:

destroys germs.

best essences:

[st] birch bud	[st] caraway seed	[st] clove bud	[s] dill
[st] juniper berry	[n] lime	[st] myrrh	[st] pine needles

elasticity – skin:

pure essential essences which are beneficial in helping retain the skins elasticity.

elasticity-essences:

[st] sweet basil	[s] benzoin	[st] carrot seed	[s] chamomiles
[s] frankencense	[s]***jasmine**	[s]***lavender**	[st] lemongrass
[s] linden blossom	[s]***mandarin**	[st] myrrh	[s] neroli
[s] rose.			

best combination: [s]***jasmine** [s]***mandarin** [s]***lavender**.

returns skin colour: [s]***tangerine**.

dry-mature-ageing skin: [s] vetivert.

puffiness: [s] celery seed [st] swt fennel seed.

wrinkles:

[st] carrot seed	[s] clary sage	[st] swt fennel seed	[s] frankencense
[n] geranium	[s] guaiacwood	[s] helichrysum	[s] jasmine
[n] lemon	[st] palmarosa	[s] patchouli	[s] rose
[st] rose geranium	[st] rosewood	[s] sandalwood	[eu] spikenard
[s] tangerine	[s] vetivert	[s] ylang-ylang.	

carrier oils:

vitamin A - **vitamin** E - **rosehip** - **sesame seed** - **jojoba** - **wheatgerm** oils.

---

emollient-agents:

are essential essences which are soothing and softening to the skin.

emollient-essences:

are soothing and softening to the skin - usually sedative actions.

[s] cedarwood atlas	[s] chamomiles	[n] geranium	[n] helichrysum
[b] hyssop	[s] immortelle	[s] jasmine	[s] lavender
[n] lemon	[s] linden blossom	[s] mandarin	[s] neroli
[s] rose	[s] sandalwood	[s] tagetes	[s] tangerine
[s] verbena, lemon.			

---

escharotic-agents:

are used for the treating and removal of warts; which are masses produced by uncontrolled growths of epithelial skin cells; a virus (**papillomavirus**) most warts are non-cancerous.

escharotic-essences:

[st]*cinnamon leaf	[st] garlic	[s] lavender	[n] lemon
[st] santolina.			

Aromatherapy treatment:

applications consist of topical application of **antiviral** essences to the wart, a thin layer of vege gel or similar non-toxic gel for preventing the concentrated pure essential essences from coming into contact with the healthy skin - cover with a bandaid, re-apply periodically.

orthodox medical treatment:

may involve **cryosurgery** with **liquid nitrogen - electrosurgery - chemical destruction - injections - carbon dioxide - laser surgery - surgical excision - or immunotherapy.**

antiviral-essences:

use **antiviral-agents** for the removal of warts.

[st] carrot seed	*castor oil	[s]*cinnamon leaf	[st] clove bud
[st]*garlic	[s] lavender	[n]*lemon	[st] onion
[st] santolina	[st] thuja	+ *castor oil...	

---

eye muscle strengthener:

essential essences which are strengthening to the muscles of the eye muscles.
suggested-essences:

| [st]*carrot | [n] lemon | [n] lime | [s] linden blossom. |

medium: **local rub**.

applications: (apply gently around the eyes - and over the eye lids gently).

---

facial-capillary-treatment:

[s] chamomile   [s] parsley herb   [s] rose.

carrier oils:

rosehip seed oil - **vitamin** E oil - make into a lotion - use as a massage (**gentle**) **2**x a day.

It will take a few weeks to notice an improvement in skin texture.

6 months before elasticity returns to capillaries - massage religiously **1**x a day - improve diet - **remove alcohol - tea - coffee - caffeine drinks - nicotine - extreme cold or cold foods** - avoid if possible or reduce to a minimum.

Do not wash face in hot water; avoid facial steaming, saunas etc.

[st]*carrot seed;   (mix with **almond** oil, restores tone and elasticity, may reduce wrinkles).

---

haemostatic-agents:

arrests bleeding or haemorrhage - essences which reduce the **blood-clotting time**.

haemostatic-essences:

essences which reduce the **blood-clotting time**.

[st] cinnamon leaf	[s] cypress	[n]*geranium	[s]*lavender
[n]*lemon	[n] lime	[s] rose	[st] rose geranium
[rub] terebinth	[st] yarrow.		

---

hair care:

treatment for excessive sebum production - use as a astringent - for cell regenerating actions - scalp problems - hair growth - greasy hair - also dandruff by reducing excessive production of sebum.

medium:

| applications: | **4** dr [s] clary sage > | **30** ml **jojoba oil** - use as a hair root stimulant. |
| | [s] cyprus; | good for adding to blends for oily hair. |

---

hair growth stimulant:

several pure essential essences are very effective in stimulating atrophied hair follicles into producing hair growth - not only that, pure essential essences (**unlike chemical drugs**) are harmless to the human being when used in correct formulation - they do not perform miracles, but they can certainly help a great deal.

It is important to realise one will be doing their hair a great service if working on the whole of the body.

The **circulatory** and **lymphatic systems** should be worked on also.

effective essences:

[**st**] rosemary	[s] neroli	[s] lavender	[**n**] geranium
[**st**] swt basil	[s] cypress	[s] sandalwood	[s] cedarwood atlas.

use these essences sparingly, or in a blend using **3** essences in an appropriate **carrier** oil, preferred carrier oil being **jojoba** or **meadowfoam** oils, excellent in cleansing blocked hair follicles.

4-6 drops > a bath, or massage the blend into scalp twice a day.

warm oil treatments maybe applied **1x** week or up to **4x** a week during initial **6** month program.

suggested-blend:

20 drops **rosemary**, 10 drops **sandalwood**, **15** drops **lavender** > 100 mls **jojoba** or **meadowfoam** oil.

2 drops of each into 90 mls of magnetised water to be used as a rinse after **shampooing** hair.

<u>suggested-essences</u>:

[s] clary sage;   (**4** drops > > **jojoba**, as a hair root stimulant).
[s] cypress;   (also a good addition to blends for oily scalps).

Use **clary sage as an **astringent** - has **cellular regenerating actions.**
* Scalp problems and hair growth, greasy hair and dandruff by reducing excessive production of sebum.

<u>hair tonic</u>:

Rub this mixture into the hair roots to stimulate hair growth.

[st]***swt basil essence** is especially effective when blended with **lavender** essence and a **sweet** type of **rosemary** called **rosemary verbenon**.

This mixture is rubbed into the hair roots to stimulate hair growth.

[s]***lavender**   +   [st]***rosemary verbenon** which is a sweet type of **rosemary**.

<u>medium</u>:

take a few drops of blended essences and using finger tips, rub into the bristles of a soft brush, brush through hair, use your finger tips to massage the hair at the roots to stimulate blood circulation, finally the hair is gently but completely brushed with the brush. Repeat this daily to clean out the hair root follicles and to stimulate hair growth - if the mixture is too strong, it may be diluted by half with **jojoba** oil, which has a reputation for dissolving the **clogging debris** from the hair root follicles allowing oxygen to get in, this further improves hair growth.

---

hydrating-agents:

helps in replacing loss of moisture to the skin tissue ie; **hydrating** of the skin which has been dehydrated for various reasons - **lack of water** - to the **weather**.

hydrating-essences:

| [**st**] palmarosa | [s] rose | [**st**] rose geranium. |

---

hypersensitivity:

A state of altered reactivity in which the body reacts with an exaggerated response to a foreign agent.

hypersensitivity-reactions are pathologic processes induced by the **immune response** and may be classified as immediate or delayed,

[1] the immediate hypersensitivity reactions (**anaphylaxis**);
[2] in which injury is produced by antibody against tissue antigens, (**nephrotoxic nephritis**);
[3] in which injury is produced by antigen-antibody complex, (**arthus reaction and serum sickness**);
[4] the delayed hypersensitivity reactions e.g; (**contact dermatitis**) to name a few.

antiallergenic-essences:

the best **antiallergenics** are listed below, these are the best, but also refer to full list of **antiallergenics**.

| [s] lavender | [s] melissa | [s]***khellin** | [s] ylang-ylang. |

insecticidal-agents:

plant essences which excel at discouraging or kills creepy crawly flying insects and pests.

insecticidal-essences:

[st] aniseed	[st] bay laurel	[s] bergamot	[st] birch bud
[st] cajeputi	[st] caraway seed	[st] cedarwood atlas	[st] cinnamon leaf
[s]***citronella**	[st] clove bud	[s] cypress	[st] eucalyptus, radiata
[st] swt fennel seed	[st] garlic	[n] geranium	[st] juniper berry
[s] lavender	[st] spike lavender	[n] lemon	[st] lemongrass
[n] lime	[st] litsea cubeba	[st] may chang	[n] myrtle
[st] niaouli	[st] origanum	[st] parsley	[s] patchouli
[st] peppermint	[st]***pennyroyal**	[st] pine needles	[st] rose geranium
[st] rosemary	[st] rosewood	[st] spearmint	[s] tagetes
[st] tea-tree	[rub] terebinth	[st] swt thyme	[s] verbena, lemon
[s] vetivert	[st] yarrow.		

mosquitos-flies:	[st] swt basil +	[st] cyprus +	[st] eucalyptus.
mosquitos-flies:	[s] bergamot +	[s] lavender.	
wasps-insect bites:	[st]***swt basil.**		
head lice-fleas-lice:	[s] cajeputi.		
insect bites-lice-ticks:	[st]***tea tree.**		
bites-snake bites:	[s] **patchouli.**		

insect repellent-agents:

plant essences which keep insects etc at bay.

repellent-essences:

[s]***bergamot**	[st] citronella	[st] clove bud	[s] cypress
[st] eucalyptus	[n] geranium	[st] galbanum	[s] lavender
[n] lemon	[st] lemongrass	[n] lime	[s] swt orange
[st]***pennyroyal**	[st] peppermint	[st] rose geranium	[st] rosemary
[st] rosewood	[st] spearmint	[st] yarrow.	

termites-ants-moths:	[s] cedarwood atlas.
keeps pests away:	[st] rose geranium.
insects-moths:	[s] vetivert.
fleas-mozzies:	[s] tagetes.
fleas-bugs-lice:	[st] pine needles.
mice-ants-cockroaches:	[st]***peppermint** + [st] eucalyptus.

---

parasiticides:

rids scabies - lice - fleas - diluted parasitic blend - by local application.

parasiticide-essences:

[st] aniseed	[st] caraway	[st] cinnamon leaf	[st] citronella
[st] clove bud	[st] cumin	[st]***eucalyptus** radiata	[st] garlic
[s] lavender	[n] lemon	[st] lemongrass	[n] myrtle
[st] origanum	[st] peppermint	[st] rose geranium	[st] rosemary
[rub] terebinth	[st] swt thyme.		

repels fleas-lice:

| [st]*eucalyptus | [n] geranium | [s] lavender | [n] lemon |
| [st]*pennyroyal | [st]*rosemary | [st]*tea tree. | |

---

penetrating-agents:

pure essential plant essences which are classified as **penetrating**, penetrate to the core of the problem.

penetrating essences:

[st] cardamom.

---

photo-toxic:

may cause skin irritation and / or pigmentation on exposure to direct sunlight.

[st]*angelica root.

---

preservative-agents:
helps in the rejuvenation of ageing skin.

| [s]*benzoin | [s] cedarwood atlas | [s]*elemi | [s]*frankencense |
| [st]*galbanum | [st]*myrrh (skin) | [s]*neroli. | |

---

prophylactic-agents:

helping to prevent Dis-ease.

prophylactic-essences:

[n] birch bud   [st] garlic   [b] hyssop   [st] lemongrass.

radiation antodote:

these pure essential plant essences intervenes with **radiation therapy**.

antidotes:

[**st**]*****yarrow**   [s] lavender.

---

rehydrating essences:

helps in replacing loss of moisture to skin tissue ie; rehydration of the skin which has been **dehydrated** for various reasons - **lack of water** - to the **weather**.

rehydrating-essences:

[s] rose   [**st**] palmarosa   [**st**] rose geranium.

---

rejuvenator-agents for skin:

rejuvenator-agents rejuvenate the skin tissue to regenerate new cell tissue.

rejuvenator-essences:

rejuvenates the skin **tissue rejuvenating** new cell tissue.

[s] benzoin	[**st**]*****carrot seed**	[s] frankencense	[s] jasmine
[s] lavender	[**n**] lemon	[**st**] myrrh	[s] neroli
[s] patchouli	[**st**] peppermint	[**b**] pettitgrain	[s] rose
[**st**] rosemary	[s] sandalwood.		

[s] ylang-ylang; > **30** mls **sweet almond** and **apricot kernel** oils.

decongestant-essences:

[st] juniper berry [s] swt orange [st] peppermint [st] pine needles
[s] patchouli [st] rosemary [st] rosewood

elasticity-essences:

rejuvenators help in retaining the skins elasticity.

[st] swt basil [s] benzoin [st] carrot seed [s] chamomiles
[s] frankencense [s]***jasmine** [s]***lavender** [st] lemongrass
[s] linden blossom [s]***mandarin** [st] myrrh [s] neroli
[s] rose.

best combination:

[s]***jasmine** [s]***mandarin** [s]***lavender**

refreshes complexion:

[s]***tangerine**

dry-mature-ageing skins:

[s] vetivert.

wrinkles:

[st] carrot seed [s] clary sage [st] swt fennel seed [s] frankencense
[n] geranium [s] guaiacwood [s] helichrysum [s] jasmine
[n] lemon [st] palmarosa [s] patchouli [s] rose
[st] rose geranium [st] rosewood [s] sandalwood [eu] spikenard
[s] tangerine [s] vetivert [s] ylang-ylang.

resolvent-agents:

are used to dissolve boils and swellings.

resolvent-essences:

[st] swt fennel seed	[st] galbanum	[st] garlic	[st] grapefruit
[b] hyssop	[st] rosemary.		

---

rubefacient-agents:

are **warming**; by increasing the blood flow – redness occurs when applied to the skin.

rubefacient-essences:

[st]***black pepper**	[st] camphor	[st]***eucalyptus** radiata	[st]***ginger**
[st]***juniper berry**	[s] swt marjoram	[st] origanum	[st] pimento
[st] pine needles	[st]***rosemary**	[rub] terebinth.	

---

skin cleanser:

an excellent skin cleansing formulation using a base of ReJuV Crème formulation – use a small quantity;

200 grams	very hot magnetised water, add
200 grams	ReJuV Crème.

<u>Mix in blender until thickens - doubles in volume - when cooled to **40c** - add;</u>

10 drops	[s] frankencense,
10 drops	[s] palmarosa,
10 drops	[**st**] niaouli,
6 drops	[**st**] lemongrass
6 drops	[s] benzoin; and mix well.

<u>skin glands</u>:

there are **3** types of glands associated with the skin; **sebaceous - sudoriferous - ceruminous**.

<u>sebaceous gland</u>:

sebaceous is an **exocrine gland** in the **dermis** of the skin - usually associated with the hair follicle, it secretes **sebum** also called oil gland - when **sebaceous glands** of the face become enlarged due to an accumulation of sebum, acne lesions develop, these are called **blackheads** - as **sebum** is nutritive to certain bacteria - boils - pimples are prone to occur. The colour of blackheads is due to melanin and oxidised oil, not dirt.

<u>blackheads – blocked skin pores</u>:

[**n**]***jojoba oil**   [**st**] cajeputi   [**st**] tea tree.

<u>sudoriferous glands</u>:

are sweat glands, these are divided into **2** principle types based on structure and location.

<u>apocrine and eccrine sweat glands</u>:

apocrine sweat glands:

are simple, branched tubular glands - their distribution is limited primarily to the skin of the **axilla, pubis** and pigmented areas (areolae) of the breasts; the secretory portion of the apocrine sweat glands is located in the dermis or subcutaneous layer and the excretory duct opens into hair follicles - these glands begin to function at puberty, produce more viscous secretion than eccrine sweat glands.

perspiration:

is the substance produced by the **sudoriferous sweat glands** - its a mixture of; **water - salts** (*mostly* NaCl) - **urea - uric acid - amino acid - ammonia - sugar - lactic acid - ascorbic acid**.

Its principal function is to help regulate body's temperature by evaporation of water in perspiration which carries off large quantities of heat energy from the body's surface, also helps to eliminate wastes.

eccrine sweat glands:

are simple - coiled - tubular glands and are much more common than **apocrine sweat glands**.

They are distributed throughout the skin except the areas of the lips - nailbeds of fingers - toes - glans - penis - glans clitoris - labia minora - eardrums.

Eccrine sweat glands are more densely situated in the palms of the hands & the soles of the feet, their density being high as **3,000** per **2.5** cm in the palm area. The secretory portion of the **eccrine sweat glands** is located in the subcutaneous layer, and the secretory duct projects upwards through the **dermis** and is **epidermis** to terminate at a pore in the surface of the epidermis. **Eccrine sweat glands** function throughout life producing a secretion that is more watery than **apocrine sweat glands**.

ceruminous:

in certain parts of the skin, **sudoriferous glands** are modified as **ceruminous glands**, such modified glands are simple, coiled tubular glands present in the external auditory meatus (canal) - the secretory portions of **ceruminous glands** lie in the subcutaneous layer, deep to sebaceous glands, and the excretory ducts open either directly onto the surface of the external auditory meatus or into ducts of sebaceous glands - the combined secretion of the **ceruminous** and **sebaceous glands** is called (*cerumen*) - cerumen, together with hairs in the external auditory meatus, provides a sticky barrier that prevents the entrance of foreign bodies - some people produce an abnormal amount of **cerumen**, or (*earwax*), in the external auditory meatus, it then becomes impacted and prevents sound waves from reaching the tympanic membrane, eardrum. The orthodox treatment for **impacted cerumen** is usually periodic ear irrigation or removal of wax with a blunt instrument by trained medical personnel.

deodourant-essences:

destroys the bacteria causing the odour.

[s] benzoin	[s]***bergamot**	[st] citronella	[s]***clary sage**
[**st**] coriander	[s]***cypress**	[**n**] geranium	[**st**]***eucalyptus radiata**
[s]***lavender**	[**st**] lemongrass	[**st**] myrrh	[s]***neroli**
[s] patchouli	[**b**]***pettitgrain**	[**st**] pine needles	[**st**]***rose geranium**
[**st**]***rosewood**...			

---

skin photosensitisation:

essences which may cause skin photosensitisation to ultra-violet rays from the sun.

photosensitisation-essences:

avoid sun exposure for at least 4 hours after using any of these essences in a massage blend.

[s] bergamot	[st] grapefruit	[n] lemon	[n] lime
[s] mandarin	[b] pettitgrain	[s] swt orange.	

---

skin-tone:

elasticity of the skin - pure essential plant essences which are beneficial in helping retain the **skins elasticity**.

elasticity-essences:

rejuvenators help in retaining the skins elasticity.

[st] swt basil	[s] benzoin	[st] carrot seed	[s] chamomiles
[s] frankencense	[s]*jasmine	[s]*lavender	[st] lemongrass
[s] linden blossom	[s]*mandarin	[st] myrrh	[s] neroli
[s] rose	[eu] spikenard.		

best combination:

[s]*jasmine   [s]*mandarin   [s]*lavender.

returns skin colour:

[s]*tangerine.

puffiness:

[s] celery seed   [st] swt fennel seed.

wrinkles:

[**st**] carrot seed	[s] clary sage	[**st**] swt fennel seed	[s] frankencense
[**n**] geranium	[s] guaiacwood	[s] helichrysum	[s] jasmine
[**n**] lemon	[s] palmarosa	[s] patchouli	[s] rose
[**st**] rose geranium	[**st**] rosewood	[s] sandalwood	[**eu**] spikenard
[s] tangerine	[s] vetivert	[s] ylang-ylang.	

carrier oils:
jojoba * vitamin A * vitamin E * rosehip * sesame seed oil * wheatgerm oils.

---

skin-types:

blemished skin:

1) course thick texture
2) generally oily shine
3) usually contains blackheads
4) may contain pimples
5) is red and uneven texture.

combination skin:

1) combination, consists 'T' area, forehead, nose, chin, are oily areas.
2) cheeks and sides of face are normal to dry skin.
3) oily area will have course texture - oily shine - enlarged pores - blackheads - whiteheads.
4) normal - dry area will have little tightness to flakiness, may have fine lines around eyes.

congested-skin-essences:

[**st**] swt basil	[s] celery seed	[s] chamomile	[s] clary sage
[**st**] eucalyptus radiata	[**st**] swt fennel seed	[**st**] juniper berry	[**n**] lemon.

oily-skin-essences:

1) course thick texture.
2) oily shine.
3) enlarges pores.
4) blackheads and whiteheads.
5) may have sallow skin.
6) an occasional blemish.

[s] amyris   [s] bergamot   [s] elemi   [s] frankencense
[st] juniper berry   [n] lemon.

dry-skin-essences:

[s] frankencense   [st] myrrh   [s] patchouli   [s] rose
[st] rosewood   [s] sandalwood   [s] vetivert.

normal-dry-skin-essences:

1) fine texture skin with NO visible pores.
2) sometimes scattered flakiness.
3) a healthy glow.
4) can have unevenness in colour and tone.
5) may have premature tiny lines around eyes and mouth.

[s] frankencense   [st] myrrh   [s] patchouli   [s] rose
[st] rosewood   [s] sandalwood   [s] vetivert.

mature-dry-skin-essences:

1) dry crepe texture with loss of elasticity and firmness
2) can be sallow - lifeless - lacking in colour and tone - or fine - fair - delicate looking.
3) pronounced expression lines and wrinkles around eyes and mouth.
4) sagging contours.

[s] clary sage	[s] cypress	[s] frankencense	[s] guaiacwood
[n] geranium	[s] helichrysum	[s] jasmine	[n] lemon
[s] linden blossom	[st] palmarosa	[s] rose geranium	[eu] spikenard.

ageing-skin-essences:

[s] clary sage	[s] cypress	[s] frankencense	[s] guaiacwood
[n] geranium	[s] helichrysum	[s] jasmine	[n] lemon
[s] linden blossom	[s] rose geranium	[eu] spikenard.	

wrinkled-skin-essences:

[st] carrot seed	[s] clary sage	[st] swt fennel seed	[s] frankencense
[n] geranium	[s] guaiacwood	[s] helichrysum	[s] jasmine
[n] lemon	[st] palmarosa	[s] patchouli	[s] rose
[st] rose geranium	[st] rosewood	[s] sandalwood	[eu] spikenard
[s] tangerine	[s] vetivert	[s] ylang-ylang.	

sensitive-skin:

1) broken capillaries.
2) highly coloured and uneven appearance.
3) often very fair and translucent skin.
4) can react to wind, sun, alcohol, by becoming red and uneven.
5) maybe any other skin types.

all type skins:

[st] angelica root.

cleansers:

| [s] chamomiles | [st] rose geranium | [s] frankencense. |

skin-cleanser:

an excellent skin cleansing blend is;

200 gr	very hot pure water.		
200 gr	ReJuV, mix in blender till thickens and doubles in quantity - when cool;		
10 drops each	[s] frankencense	[s] palmarosa	[st] niaouli
6 drops each	[st] lemongrass	[s] benzoin;	mix well.

skin-softener:

| [s] cedarwood atlas | [s] cypress | [s] frankencense. |

skin-toner:

[st] lemongrass [s] linden blossom [s] rose.

skin-tonics:

[st] angelica root.

---

styptic-agents:

essences arrests external bleeding.

styptic-essences:

[s] cypress [n] geranium [s]*lavender* [n]*lemon*
[st] rose geranium.

sudorific-agents:

use **sudorifics** to induce **sweating** - increases **perspiration** - speeds up **cleansing** - **drains fluids** - relieves **body poisons** post illnesses.

[**st**] angelica root	[**st**]***swt basil**	[**st**] bay laurel	[**st**] cajeputi
[**st**] camphor	[**st**] cardamom	[s]***chamomiles**	[**st**] cinnamon leaf
[s] dill	[**st**] swt fennel seed	[s] frankencense	[**st**] garlic
[**st**] ginger	[**b**] hyssop	[**st**]***juniper berry**	[s] lavender
[s] linden blossom	[s] melissa	[**st**] myrrh	[**st**] origanum
[**st**]***peppermint**	[**st**] pine needles	[**st**]***rosemary**	[**st**]***tea tree**.

antisudorific-essences:

use **antisudorific-essences** to reduce sweating.

[s] clary sage	[**st**] cypress	[s] elemi	[**n**] common sage.

---

tissue stimulant:

stimulates **tissue regeneration** for quick healing.

regenerator-essence:

[s]***neroli**.

---

vasoconstrictor-agents:

contraction of the blood vessel walls.

vasoconstrictor-essences:

[s] cypress   [n] geranium   [n] lemon   [st] peppermint
[st] rose geranium.

---

vasodilator-agents:

dilation of the blood vessels - excessive sports exertion - tired aching limbs.

vasodilator-essences:

[st]*black pepper   [st] garlic   [s] swt marjoram.

---

venous-tonic:

is a tonic to the veins.

tonic-essences:

[n]*lemon.

---

vulnerary:

prevent tissue degeneration, arrests bleeding in wounds enabling wounds to heal quicker.

vulnerary-essences:

vulnerary-essences help in the prevention of tissue degeneration.

[s]*benzoin	[s]*bergamot	[n]*calendula	[st] camphor
[s]*chamomiles	[s] elemi	[st]*eucalyptus radiata	[s] frankencense
[st] galbanum	[n]*geranium	[b] hyssop	[st] juniper berry

[st] lavandin	[s]*lavender	[s] swt marjoram	[st]*myrrh
[st] niaouli	[st] origanum	[st] rose geranium	[st] rosemary
[st] santolina	[st] tarragon	[st]*tea tree.	

---

weight loss:

some pure essential plant essences which are valuable in the reduction of body fats.

fat-burner-essences:

[st] swt basil	[s] bergamot	[st] black pepper	[st]*cardamom
[s] cypress	[st] **swt fennel seed**	[st] grapefruit	[st] juniper berry
[s]*lavender	[n]*lemon	[st] lemongrass	[n] lime
[s] swt orange	[st] onion	[st] origanum	[b] pettitgrain
[st] rosemary	[n] common sage	[st] swt thyme	

medium: **massage - local body rub.**

application: (best used in a massage blend and vigorous local rub to affected areas of the body).

THERAPEUTIC ESSENCES for the   (part three)   79
INTEGUMENTARY IMBALANCES:

[s] amyris	[st] angelica root	[st] aniseed	[st] swt basil	[st] bay laurel
[s] benzoin	[s] bergamot	[st] birch bud	[st] black pepper	[s] brahmi
[st] cajeputi	[st] caraway seed	[st] carrot seed	[s] cedarwood atlas	[s] celery seed
[s] chamomiles	[st] cinnamon leaf	[s] clary sage	[st] clove bud	[st] coriander

[s] cypress	[st] elemi	[st] eucalyptus radiata	[st] swt fennel seed	[s] fir needle
[s] frankencense	[st] galbanum	[st] garlic	[n] geranium	[st] ginger
[st] grapefruit	[s] guaiacwood	[s] helichrysum	[s] hypericum	[st] hyssop
[s] immortelle	[st] inula	[s] jasmine	[st] juniper berry	[st] lavandin
[s] lavender	[st] spike lavender	[n] lemon	[st] lemongrass	[n] lime
[s] linden blossom	[s] mandarin	[s] swt marjoram	[st] may chang	[s] melissa
[st] myrrh	[n] myrtle	[s] neroli	[st] niaouli	[st] swt orange
[st] origanum	[st] palmarosa	[st] parsley herb	[s] patchouli	[st] peppermint
[s] pettitgrain	[st] pimento leaf	[st] pine needles.	[st] rose geranium	[s] rose
[st] rosemary	[st] rosewood	[s] sandalwood	[st] spearmint	[s] spikenard
[s] tagetes	[s] tangerine	[st] tea tree	[st] swt thyme	[s] verbena
[s] vetivert	[s] violet leaf	[st] yarrow	[s] ylang-ylang.	

www.ingramcontent.com/pod-product-compliance
Lightning Source LLC
LaVergne TN
LVHW011726060526
838200LV00051B/3039